MOLECULAR PHARMACOLOGY:

A Short Course

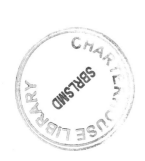
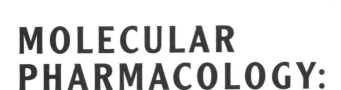

MOLECULAR PHARMACOLOGY:
A Short Course

Terry Kenakin, PhD
Principal Research Scientist
Department of Receptor Biochemistry
Glaxo Wellcome Research
Research Triangle Park, North Carolina

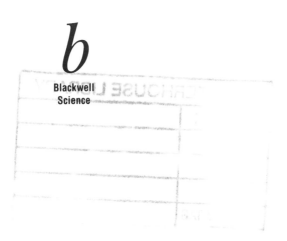

Blackwell Science

Blackwell Science

Editorial offices:

238 Main Street, Cambridge, Massachusetts
    02142, USA
Osney Mead, Oxford OX2 0E1, England
25 John Street, London WC1N 2BL, England
23 Ainslie Place, Edinburgh EH3 6AJ, Scotland
54 University Street, Carlton, Victoria 3053, Australia
Other Editorial Offices:
Arnette Blackwell SA, 224, Boulevard Saint Germain,
    75007 Paris, France
Blackwell Wissenschafts-Verlag GmbH
    Kurfürstendamm 57, 10707 Berlin, Germany
    Zehetnergasse 6, A-1140 Vienna, Austria

Distributors:

USA
Blackwell Science, Inc.
238 Main Street
Cambridge, Massachusetts 02142
(Telephone orders: 800-215-1000
    or 617-876-7000; Fax orders: 617-492-5263)

Canada
Copp Clark Professional
200 Adelaide Street, West, 3rd Floor
Toronto, Ontario M5H 1W7
(Telephone orders: 416-597-1616
    1-800-815-9417 fax: 416-597-1617)

Australia
Blackwell Science Pty., Ltd.
54 University Street
Carlton, Victoria 3053
(Telephone orders: 03-9347-0300;
    fax orders 03-9349 3016)

Outside North America and Australia
Blackwell Science, Ltd.
c/o Marston Book Services, Ltd.
P.O. Box 269
Abingdon
Oxford OX14 4YN
England
(Telephone orders: 44-01235-465500;
    fax orders 44-01235-465555)

Acquisitions: Jane Humphreys
Production: Ellen Samia
Manufacturing: Lisa Flanagan
Typeset by Northeastern Graphic Services, Inc.
Printed and bound by Courier Companies, Inc.

©1997 by Blackwell Science, Inc.
Printed in the United States of America
97 98 99 5 4 3 2 1

The Blackwell Science logo is a trade mark of Blackwell Science Ltd., registered at the United Kingdom
Trade Marks Registry

Library of Congress Cataloging-in-Publication Data
Kenakin, Terrence P.
    Molecular pharmacology: a short course / Terry
    Kenakin.
        p.   cm.
    Includes bibliographical references and index.
    ISBN 0-86542-540-X
    1. Molecular pharmacology.   I. Title
    [DNLM: 1. Drug Design. 2. Dose-Response
        Relationship, Drug
    3. Receptors, Drug—physiology. 4. Biological
        Markers. QV 744
    K33m 1996]
    RM301.65.K459 1996
    615'. 19—dc21
    DNLM/DLC
    for Library of Congress   6-39098
                                            CIP

Biologic Systems and Definitions of Terms

I N THIS first chapter, concepts, terms, and major ideas repeatedly found in pharmacology are introduced. Section 1.1 outlines the origins of the discipline (from physiology), and section 1.2 defines biologic units, an idea expanded on in section 1.3 with the discussion of operational receptors, the basic unit on which drugs act. In section 1.4, the observed activity of drugs is delineated into the two characteristic properties of all drugs, affinity and efficacy. It is the ability to quantify these properties that allows drugs to be discovered and studied in one kind of biologic system and used in another (i.e., they are system-independent and predictive). Section 1.4 also defines the common labels given to drugs based on observed efficacy and potency.

Section 1.5 discusses the classification of biologic systems and section 1.6 the classification of drugs. This latter process is incontravertibly linked to the discovery of new drugs. Finally, section 1.7 addresses a very important tenet in pharmacology—namely the fact that drugs are selective, not specific, and that specific activity is linked to concentration and selectivity windows. These ideas are revisited in the synopsis of the chapter, section 1.8. The ideas in this chapter set the stage for the next step in pharmacology, use of the dose-response curve.

1.1 AIMS OF PHARMACOLOGIC CLASSIFICATION

The goal of this book is to present the methods devised within the science of pharmacology to discover biologic information encoded in molecules and to use this information to classify and probe biologic systems. The quest for drugs to cure disease is as old as recorded history. For example, the ancient medical papyrus edited by Georg Ebers (early dynasties of ancient Egypt) states, "...empty the belly and make all evil that is in the body of man come out..." Similarly, the study of biologic systems has been a science for many hundreds of years, and both endogenous and foreign chemicals have been used throughout this period to perturb biologic systems in order to learn more about how they function.

Approximately 150 years ago, a subculture of physiologists became more interested in the probes than in the systems and thus began tailoring their experiments to ask questions in reverse (i.e., not from the point of view of using the molecules to yield information about the physiology of the system, but rather from the point of view of using the system to yield information about the molecules). The concept of not only *finding* the most appropriate molecule for the treatment of the disease, but also of determining how to *improve* that molecule, was operative. From these beginnings, the science of *pharmacology* has borrowed from the principles of chemistry, physics, genetics, and cellular biology to form a framework for the description of molecular interaction with biologic systems.

Clearly, the most straightforward approach to finding new drugs would be the direct testing of molecules in the human host under the particular pathologic conditions targeted. This direct approach is precluded for obvious reasons. The alternatives dominate the science of pharmacology—namely, the discovery, modification, care, and treatment of biologic systems for the express purpose of measuring the biologic activity of drugs.

This book will discuss two scientific approaches. The first is the use of known drugs to classify biologic systems (referred to as *systems taxonomy*; Fig 1-1) . These procedures are used in physiology, biochemistry, and genetics. A second general approach is the use of characterized biologic systems to classify molecules (referred to as *chemical taxonomy*, see Fig 1-1). This latter process is the basis of pharmacology, medicinal chemistry, and drug discovery. For both of these endeavors, molecular estimates are needed that do not depend on the specifics of the procedures used to obtain them. Figure 1-1

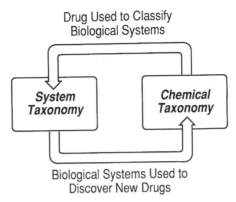

FIGURE 1-1. *The interconnected disciplines used for the discovery of new drug entities (chemical taxonomy, including pharmacology, and medicinal chemistry) and the classification of biologic systems with drugs (system taxonomy, encompassing biochemistry, physiology, and genetics).*

illustrates the essential circularity of the processes of drug and system classification.

1.2 DRUGS AND BIOLOGIC SYSTEMS

Biologic systems will refer to the responding units used to measure drug activity. Minimally, these are composed of a mechanism to recognize *stimulus* (usually chemical stimulus in the form of drugs) and to respond to that stimulus. They can be extremely simple (i.e., isolated proteins, pieces of cell membrane) or highly complex (as in whole cells, pieces of structured tissue, whole tissues, or the whole body). There are specific advantages to using any one of these systems; therefore, the choice of system often will involve the question of what information is required, which is discussed more extensively in Chapter 6.

Drugs are unique chemicals that selectively interact with biologic systems. They can *stimulate* the system and produce an increase in physiologic function, they can *depress* physiologic function, or they can have *no direct effect* on the system but *modulate the effect of other drugs*. If the interaction between two drugs is via separate targets, it is considered a functional interaction and not easily modeled by mathematic equations describing drug-receptor kinetics. If the drugs interact at the same target, there are a number of models which can be used to describe the interaction, and quantify the molecular properties of the drugs and the targets (Fig 1-2).

The questions to be considered here are these: What are the properties of a given drug molecule on a biologic system, and which of those properties are likely to be unique to the molecular structure of that drug and thus be

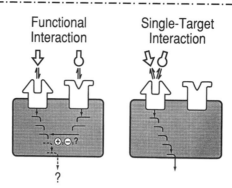

FIGURE 1-2. *Functional versus single-target drug interactions. Whereas functional stimuli can join anywhere in the stimulus-response cascade of a cell, single-target effects stem from drug interaction at the same receptor.*

transferable to other biologic systems? Such activity begins at the biologic target for that molecule.

1.3 BIOLOGIC TARGETS: OPERATIONAL RECEPTORS

This book will consider biologic targets operationally as *receptors*. These can take on many forms in cells and, in general, they have two functions: the *recognition* of molecules and the *transduction* of the information encoded in those molecules to the cell. Basically, any structure that exists to recognize chemicals (or, in the case of rhodopsin, light) and respond to that recognition qualifies operationally as a receptor. A number of procedures, able to quantify drug activity on receptors are not affected by the nature of the receptor; this allows for operational approaches to the study of drug activity.

An operational approach treats the receptor as a black box that is switched on or off to varying degrees by drugs. The molecular mechanisms by which this happens vary with different receptors, and the understanding of these mechanisms changes with the state of technology. Therefore, approaches based on knowledge of the molecular mechanism of drugs often are limited. However, once the box is switched on or off, many biologic processes deal with the signal in the same way, and the methods of quantifying activity are common to many receptors. Therefore, it is possible to transcend the molecular nature of receptor mechanism and to classify drugs and biologic systems with various pharmacologic procedures.

The other advantage to viewing the receptor for drugs as a black box is its modular nature. Receptors are the first line of interaction of biologic systems with chemicals and therefore are common throughout the body; that is, they must recognize universal chemicals, hormones, neurotransmitters. Thus, they can be considered a module that interacts with a series of host systems (Fig 1-3).

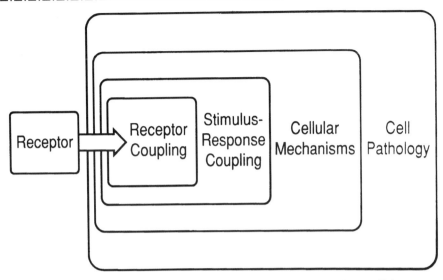

FIGURE 1-3. *Receptor molecules in layered biologic systems. The receptor is inserted into cellular systems that are themselves a collection of interactive modules. The cellular response resulting from receptor activation is the product of these processes.*

Those host systems are composed of a receptor coupling mechanism, a stimulus-response coupling mechanism, various cellular mechanisms, and often, in the case of new drug discovery, a pathologic process overlaid on the whole system. Because receptors are the first line of interaction, they frequently are studied in isolation to gain selectivity in effect and also to negate the complicating modulation of the aforementioned processes on receptors. Heterologous receptor expression systems are created genetically, with human receptors in surrogate cell lines (see Chapter 4). An operational approach to the study of receptors fits in well with this concept as it treats the receptor as a responding unit irrespective of its host.

Receptors are very specialized structures in biologic systems. They allow for extraordinary specificity in drug recognition (i.e., the slightest change in chemical structure can result in 100-fold decreases in activity) and extraordinary potency. For example, one-hundredth of a millionth (10^{-8}) of a person's weight in insulin is sufficient to prevent a life-threatening diabetic coma. In terms of area, assuming the Earth were a single cell, the receptor for the neurotransmitter acetylcholine occupies the space of the island of Jamaica, yet this area can completely control cellular function to neuronally released acetylcholine.

Cells use many structures including *ion channels, enzymes, carriers,* and a specific class of protein molecules also named *receptors,* to sense their environment and respond to it (see Fig 1-4). A distinction should be made between the conceptual idea of receptors and the specific protein structure

Extracellular Space

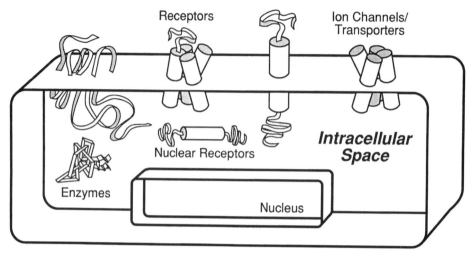

FIGURE 1-4. *Schematic diagram of a cell with approximate location of various targets for drug action.*

called *receptors*. Examples of these potential targets are given in Table 1-1. From the point of view of therapeutic intervention, these targets take in nutrients, sense chemical environments, modify nutrients, expel waste products, and generally affect the function of cells.

The various biologic targets mediate functions of biologically relevant molecules in the normally functioning cell in different ways. For example, a given enzyme may degrade a metabolic product in a cell; in this case, the endogenous ligand (the metabolic product) is modified by the target. Hor-

TABLE 1-1   Biologic Targets to Alter Cell Function

Target	Example
Receptors	G-protein coupled receptors (adrenergic)
	Direct ligand-gated channels (nicotinic acetylcholine)
	Tyrosine kinase-linked (insulin)
	Nuclear receptors (estrogen)
Ion Channels	Ca^{++}, Na^+, Cl^-
Enzymes	Acetylcholinesterase
	Angiotensin-converting
	DNA polymerase
Carriers	Norepinephrine uptake
	Serotonin uptake

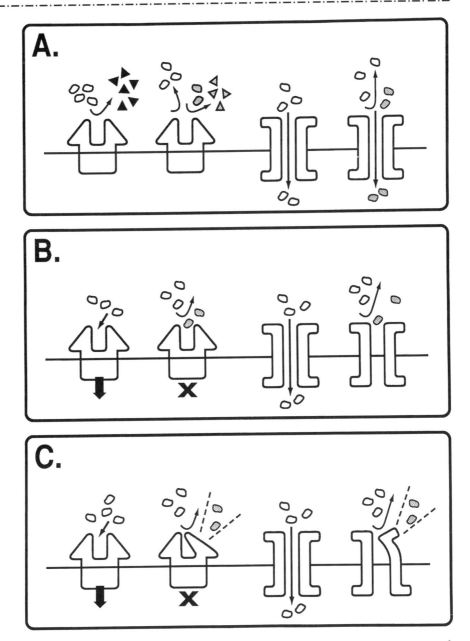

FIGURE 1-5. *Types of drug interaction at receptors. A. The drug (gray particles) becomes a surrogate for the endogenous substance acting either at a receptor (left) or at a channel transporter (right). B. Chemical interference with the drug not acting as a surrogate but rather interacting at the binding site for the endogenous receptor activator. C. Drugs bind to an accessory site on the receptor to modulate receptor action with endogenous activator.*

mone receptors, such as that for epinephrine, mediate cellular responses to hormones and do not chemically modify their ligands. Carriers translocate their ligands into different compartments.

Drugs can interact with these various targets in three general ways (Fig 1-5). The first is by acting as a surrogate for endogenous primary ligands. For example, a drug may be a false substrate for an enzyme and thus interfere with its normal metabolic function. In this case, the drug is chemically modified by the process. The same can be true for carriers in that the drug may act as a false passenger and again be removed from the reaction by virtue of being translocated into an inaccessible compartment.

The second general drug-target interaction is by chemical interference at the active site but with failure to function as a surrogate for the endogenous ligand. Thus, a drug may bind to the active site and modify metabolic function of an enzyme but also not be chemically modified by that enzyme. Similarly, a drug may block a carrier process but not be translocated by that process. Drugs that interact at the site on the biologic target where the endogenous ligand is located can be considered *competitive* drugs.

In the third type of interaction, termed *allotopic,* the drug modifies target function by binding to a site distinct from that of the endogenous ligand. It is well known that proteins and nucleic acids have delicate structures that depend on a concert of interactions between chemical groupings. Interference with some of these can disrupt the total structure of the target and thus modify ligand interaction with the target at a site distinct from that of the disruption.

1.4 SYSTEM-INDEPENDENT PROPERTIES OF DRUGS

Because receptors are designed both to recognize molecules and to transmit messages from those molecules, the act of binding of a drug to a receptor may well change the behavior of that receptor toward the cellular host. The chemical property that causes the drug to remain associated with the receptor is known as *affinity* whereas the property of the drug that causes the receptor to change its behavior toward the host is known as *efficacy.* These two drug properties are molecular in nature (i.e., inherent in the chemical structure of the drug) and, once characterized, should be constant throughout the spectrum of different biologic hosts housing that particular receptor. It follows, therefore, that if the affinity and efficacy of a particular drug can be characterized for a human receptor in a surrogate system, the result will be a valuable predictor of that drug's activity for humans in the therapeutic arena.

A cohesive structure for the understanding of drug action begins at these core molecular properties of drugs, affinity and efficacy. It will be seen repeatedly in this book that these molecular properties are expressed in complex biologic systems in a multitude of ways and that reliance on the expression of these activities, rather than on the chemical nature of these activities, can result in dissimulation and chaos.

1.4.1 Affinity

Chemicals reside in a world of energy levels. Drugs will associate themselves near a body if the energy environment for that association is better than not being near the body. Furthermore, they exist at distances away from that body according to the strengths of the interactions of chemical groupings on the molecule and on the body. These ideas are described by the chemical concept of *affinity*. The closeness of the association of a drug near the body (i.e., a protein receptor) is called *binding*.

The chemical structure of a drug gives it a presentation of energy to the receptor, which is complementary to a specific site on the receptor. Chemical forces such as ion-ion, ion-dipole, dipole-dipole, hydrogen, and Van der Waals interactions keep the drug fixed at a specific distance from the receptor with an energy of interaction. Molecules have kinetic energy from thermal agitation that periodically surpasses the energy holding the drug at the receptor; therefore, a tug-o'-war ensues in which drugs become entrapped by energy fields and are associated and then escape those fields and become dissociated from the receptor. This stochastic process of binding, dissociation, and re-binding should be considered in all aspects of drug action: Drugs do not simply stick to receptors and stay there. This idea is an essential idea to the concept of competitive drug interaction (i.e., one drug may occupy a receptor previously occupied and temporarily vacated by another).

The magnitude of the affinity between a drug and a receptor is graded by the *equilibrium dissociation constant* of the complex formed between the drug and the receptor. It is defined as the ratio of the rate of offset of the drug from the receptor divided by the rate of onset of a drug to a receptor. The reaction between a drug A and a receptor R can be described by the following scheme:

$$A + \underset{(1-y)}{R} \overset{k_1}{\underset{k_2}{\rightleftharpoons}} \underset{y}{A \cdot R} \qquad [1.1]$$

where the drug-receptor complex is denoted by $A \cdot R$. If the fraction of $A \cdot R$ produced by concentration A is y, then the remaining unbound receptor is given by $(1 - y)$. The rate of formation of $A \cdot R$ is given by the first order rate equation $k_1 A(1 - y)$ while the rate of destruction of $A \cdot R$ is given by $k_2 y$. At equilibrium, the rate of formation of $A \cdot R$ equals the rate of destruction of $A \cdot R$:

$$k_1 A(1 - y) = k_2 y \qquad [1.2]$$

Under these circumstances, the fraction of receptor occupied by the drug can be given by a rearrangement of Equation 1.2:

$$y = \frac{[A]}{[A] + k_2/k_1} \qquad [1.3]$$

The ratio of k_2/k_1 is defined as the *equilibrium dissociation constant* of the drug-receptor complex and denoted as K_{eq}. There is a physical meaning to K_{eq} in that it is the concentration of drug A that occupies 50% of the existing receptor population (i.e., $y = 0.5$). This can be shown as follows:

$$y = 0.5 = \frac{[A]}{[A] + K_{eq}} \qquad [1.4]$$

which rearranges to $[A] = K_{eq}$. Thus it can be seen that the lower the magnitude of K_{eq}, the lower the concentration of the drug needed to occupy 50% of the receptors. Therefore, the drug must have a high affinity for a low concentration to associate selectively with the receptor. For 50% receptor occupation of a drug with a K_{eq} of 10^{-8} M, for example, 10^{-8} M drug would have to be present in the receptor compartment. In contrast, if the K_{eq} of another drug were 10^{-10} M, 50% occupation would require only one-hundredth the concentration required of the first drug (10^{-10} M). Thus the drug with K_{eq} of 10^{-10} M has 100-fold more potency than the drug with a K_{eq} of 10^{-8} M.

The K_{eq} is a convenient chemical term for the various pharmacologic procedures employed to estimate drug parameters. However, it is an inverse value in that a high affinity is denoted by a very low K_{eq}. For this reason, biologists periodically use the reciprocal of K_{eq}, termed the *equilibrium association constant* or the *affinity constant* ($K_{aff} = 1/K_{eq}$). Although this is becoming less common, it is the approach of choice for mathematic modeling of receptor systems because they allow for microscopic reversibility, making manageable the manipulation of thermodynamic conservation equations (see Chapter 3).

1.4.2 Intrinsic Efficacy

Once a drug binds to a receptor, that receptor may change its behavior toward the host. The drug property that causes this to happen is termed *intrinsic efficacy*. The word intrinsic connotes its molecular nature. A common usage of the word efficacy is often to denote the particular activity of a drug in a given system. This use of the word efficacy should be differentiated from the strictly molecular description of drug activity.

Intrinsic efficacy has a scale from positive to negative, and the expression of this drug property depends very much upon the constitutive basal activity of the cell. A drug with positive efficacy is called an *agonist* and will activate receptors to promote cellular response. Similarly, a drug with negative efficacy will bind to receptors to decrease basal receptor activity; such drugs are called *inverse agonists.*

The blockade of receptor response induced by an agonist is referred to as *antagonism* and drugs that have this property are called *antagonists.* It should be recognized that antagonism is not an exclusive property of drugs; some drugs that produce response also can antagonize responses to stronger drugs.

Agonists produce an initial stimulus to a receptor that then is processed by the stimulus-response mechanisms of the system into an observable response. This usually results in amplification of the initial signal. Variation in the amplification results from variation in the efficiency of the relationship between receptor stimulus and tissue response. The molecular property of intrinsic efficacy determines the initial strength of the receptor stimulus. If this is considered to be a given mass placed on one end of a scale (Fig 1-6), the displacement of the other end of the scale would represent the resulting tissue response. The vantage point for viewing that displacement determines its magnitude. Placement of the sight line for observing the tissue response can be considered a measure of the efficiency of stimulus-response coupling. As seen in Figure 1-6, tissue I is poorly coupled, tissue II more efficiently

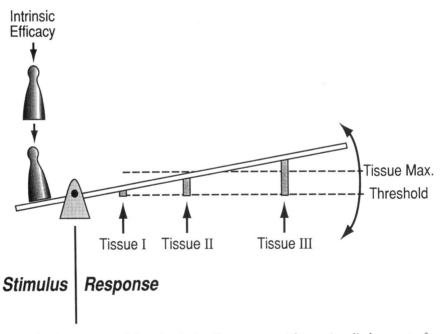

FIGURE 1-6. *The molecular property of drug intrinsic efficacy as a weight causing displacement of a lever. The arc transcribed by the opposite end of the lever represents the amplified cellular response to the receptor stimulus. The three vantage points (tissues I, II, III) represent cellular systems of increasing amplification power.*

coupled, and tissue III highly coupled in terms of the efficiency of translation of receptor stimulus into tissue response.

Agonism is further characterized in terms of the magnitude of response produced. Biologic systems produce graded increased response to drugs up to a tissue maximum, which is the maximal response that can be elicited by any drug activating a particular receptor. Two maxima need to be considered in biologic testing. The first is the maximal response that a drug can produce from a target, which is determined by the molecular structure of the drug. The second is the maximal response that the particular biologic system can produce. Thus, the drug maximum is filtered through the tissue maximum process. Drugs with different capabilities for producing the maximal stimulus from a receptor may still produce the same observable maximal response from the tissue if the drug maximum surpasses the tissue maximum (Fig 1-7). For this reason, reliance on tissue maxima to ascribe molecular properties to drugs is erroneous.

Drugs that elicit the tissue maximum response are referred to as *full agonists*. Drugs that produce a maximal response that is lower than the tissue maximum response are called *partial agonists*. In the sense that a partial agonist is weaker than a full agonist, a partial agonist can antagonize the response to a full agonist if present at an appropriate concentration. To be classified completely as a partial agonist, a drug must 1) produce a maximal response that is lower than the tissue maximum and 2) be able to antagonize a full agonist.

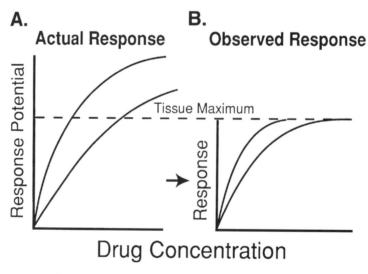

FIGURE 1-7. *Diagram representing increasing tissue response to increasing drug concentrations. A. The molecular stimulus to two drugs of differing power. B. The observed cellular response in a system that imposes a ceiling on response. The observed maximal response to the two drugs of differing power is the same.*

TABLE 1-2 Expression of Drug Efficacy

Molecular Property	Expression in System	Classification
Positive efficacy	Produces tissue maximal response	Full agonist
	Produces sub-maximal response	Partial agonist
	Produces no direct response	Antagonist
Zero efficacy	Produces no direct response	Antagonist
Negative Efficacy	Produces no direct response	Antagonist
	Depresses basal tissue response	Inverse agonist

It will be seen in subsequent chapters that biologic systems amplify and modulate drug response to a large extent. A particular drug may be strong enough to produce a full tissue response in one system and only a partial maximal response in another. Similarly, a partial agonist in one system may be an antagonist that produces no direct response in another. Therefore, the labels *agonist, partial agonist,* and *antagonist* are *system-dependent* and not necessarily molecular properties. In fact, they are tissue-translated expressions of the molecular properties of affinity and efficacy. Consequently, it is unreliable to depend on tissue classifications of drugs (e.g., agonist, antagonist etc.). Instead, drugs must be classified in terms of the molecular properties of affinity and efficacy. The various expressions of efficacy in different biologic systems and the resulting tissue classification of the drugs are shown in Table 1-2.

Whereas the affinity between a drug and a receptor can readily be described in chemical terms, the efficacy of a drug is much more difficult to describe because numerous possible mechanisms exist for a bound drug to affect receptor function. Understanding the mechanism of efficacy is the essence of pharmacology and is a great frontier in drug research. The general mechanisms of efficacy are described in Chapter 6.

1.5 CLASSIFICATION OF BIOLOGIC SYSTEMS (Biologic Taxonomy)

A major use of drugs is in the taxonomy of biologic systems, where drugs can be used as probes of cellular processes. If the probe is characterized suitably, then its behavior in the biologic system can be used to deduce similarities between systems and thus classify a new system as either a subset of an already known one, or a totally new system. One of the most frequent examples of this is the classification of receptors into *subtypes*.

One way in which various organs exert control over their environment and function is by producing structural and functional subtypes for general classes of targets that have specific properties useful in their particular environment. For example, while there is a general class of receptors for the hormones epinephrine and norepinephrine, there are subtypes of this receptor distributed in different organs that respond differently to drugs.

An important logic involved in biologic classification relates to the failure of negative evidence to provide proof of a hypothesis. This can be illustrated by the following example: In the early years of adrenergic receptor pharmacology, the prototype antagonists were relatively equiactive on the adrenergic receptors of the lung and the heart. Though this might be taken to be presumptive evidence that the receptors in the two tissues are the same, this cannot be assumed to be the case. In fact, selective antagonists for these receptors indeed were found some years later that indicated that the receptors were subtypes and different from each other. As stated by the eminent statistician DJ Finney, "To consider that certain observations do not disprove a hypothesis does not amount to proof of a hypothesis..." It may be that there simply has not yet been negative evidence generated to disprove the hypothesis.

Clearly biologic systems can be extremely complex and sometimes not amenable to simple model and hypothesis testing. However, it is incumbent on scientists to begin with the simplest hypothesis possible that is sufficient to account for experimental data and to use this as the working hypothesis. As just discussed, hypotheses can never be proven correct (i.e., supporting evidence is only consistent with a hypothesis) but rather can only be proved incorrect. Experiments must be designed to furnish data to disprove a hypothesis. Therefore, although invocation of a new drug property (i.e., a discovered selectivity) or a new biologic pathway most likely would always explain complex data, datasets should be discussed with the most simple models until such time as the data cannot be explained in this manner. One of the most common areas in which this is encountered is the discovery of selective drug action, which suggests the discovery of a new subtype of a known receptor. Before this can be a viable alternative, the explanation of drug selectivity must be inconsistent with the existing, and simpler, hypothesis.

The tendency to weigh the body of evidence in the process of classification should be discouraged. Evidence consistent with a hypothesis cannot be weighed equally with that disproving a hypothesis. For instance, if a large sample of drug types may show two biologic processes to be equivalent, but this is negated by the observation of a single drug that shows them to be different. The equivalence is circumstantial evidence for equality; the exception reveals the difference.

As drugs with known characteristics are used to probe unknown biologic systems, the databank usually aims the researcher toward grouping the process into an already known category. This is appropriate until data is generated that does not allow the common classification and, when this occurs, a new category is classified.

Finally, as illustrated in Figure 1-1, the essentially circular nature of the classification process should not be forgotten. Specifically, all classifications of biologic systems with drugs are based on the assumed classification of the probes (drugs) used to study them. If these assumed properties are erroneous, then all ensuing classifications with that probe will also be erroneous. For example, if drug A is assumed, mistakenly, to be subtype X–selective, then as drug A is used in unknown biologic systems and found to be active, this activity may be falsely ascribed to process subtype X. This has a cascading effect in that every process of chemical taxonomy with the biologic process (i.e., testing of the effects of new molecules on the biologic system) is in danger of being incorrect: Active molecules will falsely be described as sub-type process X–selective as well. This illustrates the importance of pharma-cologic (chemical) taxonomy.

1.6 THE DISCOVERY OF NEW DRUGS (Chemical Taxonomy)

The second major process in biologic research is the use of biologic systems to discover unique chemicals to be used for therapy. The aim is to quantify molecular properties of chemicals that herald useful therapeutic activity. In the process of drug discovery, medicinal chemists require data on new chemi-cal entities to improve on activity and these data cannot depend on particular biologic testing systems. Thus, medicinal chemists cannot use statements about activity such as, "the compound is active in the COS-7 transfected cell but not active in the HEK 293 transfected cell." What are required are meth-ods to measure the activity of molecules in *chemical* terms. These terms then transcend biologic testing systems so that activity will be predictable in hu-mans. It is hoped that the estimates of drug activity will be sufficiently hardy to be useful in systems modified by pathology.

A therapeutically useful drug must have certain properties that often are not found in the same molecule. Therefore, a "lead" molecule that possesses the primary activity of interest must first be found to serve as a template on which medicinal chemists can build the other required properties. In order of increasing discovery potential, the required properties of therapeutic drugs are given in Table 1-3.

The drug discovery process is structured such that the order of quantifi-cation of these properties is similar to the order in which they are listed in the table. The various biologic assays required to detect these properties are all different and parallel the order of discovery with increasing complexity. Thus, the discovery process can be viewed as a series of steps, each dependent on the previous one (Fig 1-8). It can be seen from Figure 1.8 that the population of

TABLE 1-3   Properties of Therapeutic Drugs in Order of Increasing Discovery Potential

Affinity	Binds the drug to the target
Efficacy	Modifies target when appropriate
Favorable kinetics	Must have a reasonable rate of onset to be effective within a useful time frame
	Must have a rate of offset from the molecular target to allow control of concentration
	No long-term accumulation unless especially required
Chemical stability	Not subject to spontaneous changes in chemical structure
Metabolic stability	Not vulnerable to degradative enzymes and/or biologic uptake systems
Bioavailability	Must be able to reach molecular target by the chosen route of administration (i.e., orally active drug must be absorbed from the gastrointestinal tract and delivered to the bloodstream)
Favorable toxicology	Must have a useful therapeutic window (i.e., as large a margin as possible between minimally active dose and minimally toxic dose)
	Toxicity to be minimal

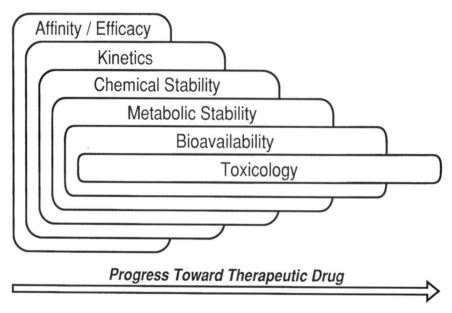

FIGURE 1-8. *The required properties of new therapeutic entities represented as increasing levels of stringency. The relative size of the boxes reflects the usual diminution of active samples fulfilling the requirements.*

molecules of interest dwindles during this process. Whereas a series of molecules all may contain the primary activity of interest, fewer will have the
required concert of activities needed for a useful therapeutic drug.

The most difficult step is discovery of a molecule with primary activity
at the molecular target (i.e., so-called lead discovery). This is because, while
a great deal of prior art and information usually is available to enhance
properties of molecules once they are discovered (i.e., there are many known
procedures to change metabolically unstable chemical groups into metabolically stable ones), the discovery of novel chemical entities often has no
rational starting point. Therefore, the screening for new drugs becomes a
sampling problem. The relevant populations are the complete library of all
possible chemical structures and the complete library of all possible biologic
systems. The process begins by sampling the population of biologic systems
to determine the appropriate target, which is a two-step process. The first
involves the testing of standard drugs chosen from chemical space (step 1,
Fig 1-9). The second involves the fine tuning of the biologic system so
that it is robust and appropriate for drug testing.

Once the biologic target is identified, the procedure re-enters chemical
space and begins to sample different chemical structures to try to determine
initial affinity and efficacy (see Fig 1-9). There are modeling methods that can
estimate various energy configurations of different structures; thus, an initial

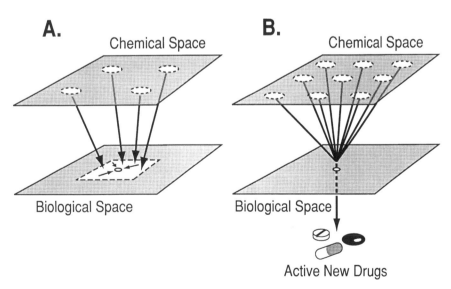

FIGURE 1-9. *The process of new drug discovery. A. Characterized drugs from chemical space are used to characterize a biologic system. B. Once the appropriate biologic system is identified, as large a sampling as possible is made from chemical space and is screened for new drug activity.*

screen may consider as diverse a sampling of structures as possible to try to cover the maximum number of possibilities. When a compound possessing affinity (and, if appropriate, efficacy) for the biologic test system is found, two processes begin. In one, a sampling of similar structures is tested along with chemical modifications of the original compound to enhance activity. In the second process the lead compound and subsequent leads are subjected to different tests to determine suitability according to the other requirements of a therapeutic drug listed in Table 1-3.

1.7 SELECTIVITY AND SPECIFICITY

Drugs are characterized and labeled by their most prominent activity, not their only activity. In general, drugs can have effects on many biologic systems and must be used within concentration limits to achieve selectivity. For example, Figure 1-10 shows the concentrations at which the drug yohimbine interacts with various biologic receptors. It can be seen from this figure that, although yohimbine is an antagonist of α_2-adrenergic receptors at concentrations lower than those needed to activate other receptors, at higher concen-

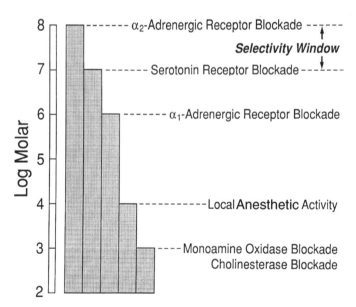

FIGURE 1-10. *Bar graph showing the negative logarithm for the molar potency (equilibrium dissociation constants) of yohimbine on various biologic systems. At concentrations greater than 10^{-8} M, yohimbine interacts with α_2-adrenergic receptors. At 10-fold higher concentrations (10^{-7} M), yohimbine interacts with serotonin receptors. Therefore, the selectivity window for yohimbine is between these two concentrations for selective α_2-adrenergic receptor activity.*

trations it also interacts with serotonin, α_1-adrenergic receptors, and the enzymes monoamine oxidase and cholinesterase.

Drugs often are referred to as *specific*, but this term usually is not applicable to most drugs as it implies a single activity for a given biologic system. Specific activity within a given concentration range, or *selectivity* usually is more accurate. Thus, as seen in Figure 1-10, yohimbine is a selective α_2-adrenergic receptor antagonist (specific between the concentrations of 10 and 100 nM).

Yohimbine is used primarily as an α_2-adrenergic receptor blocker and commonly, the tacit assumption is made that all effects of yohimbine are due to this most prominent activity. This assumption is made regarding most drugs used in biologic experimentation, and it is a useful assumption to challenge when a unique drug effect is encountered, because overall biologic effects of drugs are often a result of a mixture of activities. Ignorance of the other properties of drugs forces conclusions based on only the most prominent activity, which can lead to potential error.

One scenario in which this ignorance of a drug's multiple properties may be a problem is in the classification of biologic systems. It is commonplace to create human biologic receptor systems with molecular biology (see Chapter 4). Thus, human receptors are transfected through genetic engineering into surrogate cells and are used for drug testing. Inevitably, the question is asked: How similar are these created systems to the natural one? Usually, a series of drugs with known activity on the natural system is tested on the genetically engineered system and the results are correlated. Figure 1-11A shows a hypothetical correlation of affinities for seven antagonists on the natural and transfected receptor system. Suitability of the transfected system is judged based on the degree of correlation—that is, whether the numbers are the same, or at least whether the relative order of the potencies is the same, in which case the system is considered a useful mimic of the natural one. However, if the correlation shows deviance, it might be supposed that the genetic manipulations have introduced another variable into the receptor system and that therefore, it is not a good model of the natural one. The tacit assumption made in these correlations is that the drugs are all *equivalent* and that their most prominent activity is the only one being expressed in these two systems. As seen in Figure 1-11A, the antagonists C, E and F are relative outliers in that they are more active in the natural system than they are on the surrogate one. On the basis of the overall correlation (and the unequal weight of data), the conclusion could be drawn that the genetically created system is not a good model for the natural one. However, if antagonists C, E and F have secondary properties that enhance their activities on that natural system, and these properties cannot be expressed in the surrogate system, then an error will have been made. Under these circumstances, antagonists E and F need to

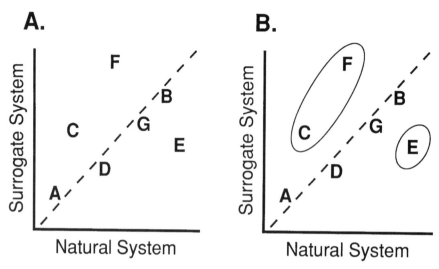

FIGURE 1-11. *Correlations of the potencies of seven drugs on two biologic systems. A. Correlation for all the drugs; line represents complete identity. B. If drugs C, E, and F are recognized to have obscuring properties on one of the systems, then the correlation of potencies changes. Whereas A suggests a poor correlation, B leads to the opposite conclusion.*

be taken out of the correlation (Fig 1-11B); the tacit assumption of equivalence of drugs cannot be supported.

Finally, it should be recognized that all uses of drugs in biologic systems, and the conclusions drawn from such uses are based on assumptions. These should be clearly understood as, in many cases, they are not directly verifiable. Therefore, when experimental data do not coincide with the hypothesis being tested, these assumptions should be examined, to determine whether they are the cause of the discrepancy. The assumptions made in the analytic procedures described in this book will be discussed within each chapter.

1.8 SYNOPSIS

The following ideas were presented in this chapter:

- There is an interdependence between the processes of using drugs to classify biologic systems and the use of those systems to discover new drugs.

- Receptors can be treated operationally as recognition and transduction units in cells.

- Receptors can be specialized membrane proteins, intracellular proteins, enzymes, or transporter channels.

- Drugs can act as surrogates for endogenous molecules, can interfere chemically with the action of endogenous molecules at the same recognition site, or can bind to separate (allotopic) sites on the receptor to otherwise modulate endogenous activity.

- Drugs have two properties, affinity and efficacy.

- The expression of efficacy can be completely dominated by the system housing the receptor (i.e., systems effects can suppress efficacy).

- Drugs often are characterized by their effects in a particular system although these effects can change with the system. The range of activities are full agonist, partial agonist, antagonist, and inverse agonist.

- Affinity is defined by an equilibrium dissociation constant.

- Classifications of receptors and drugs result from disproof of the null hypothesis.

- Drugs are always selective, but rarely specific; therefore, therapeutic windows depend on control of drug concentration.

FURTHER READING

Black JW. Receptors in the future. Postgrad Med J 1981;57:110–112.

Black JW, Jenkinson DH, Gerskowitch VP, eds. Receptor biochemistry and methodology, vol. 6. New York: Alan Liss, 1987:1–280.

Kenakin TP. Drug and organ selectivity: similarities and differences. In: Testa B, ed. Advances in drug research, vol. 15. New York: Academic, 1985:71–109.

Dose-Response Curves

THIS CHAPTER discusses the construction and use of the common currency of pharmacology, namely dose-response curves. The relationship between known independent variables and observed dependent variables results in a line possessing a maximal asymptote, slope, and location along the concentration axis (potency; section 2.1). Because individual data can vary, it often is advantageous to model the relationship mathematically to decrease bias (section 2.2). Various models use the technique of nonlinear curve fitting, and the resulting curves can be compared to theoretic models found in drug receptor theory. The most powerful use of dose-response curves involves null methods (section 2.3). These ideas are summarized further in section 2.4.

2.1 DOSE-RESPONSE CURVES

All measures of drug activity or system sensitivity come from dose-response curves. *Dose-response curve* is a general term for a graphic representation of

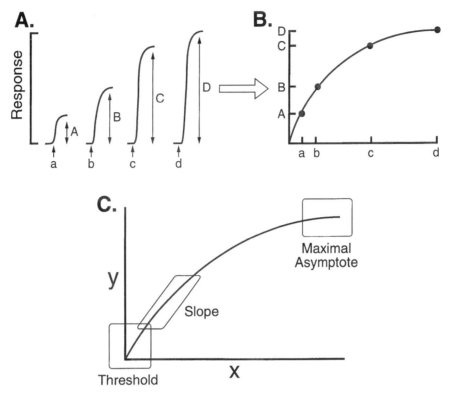

FIGURE 2-1. *The construction of dose-response curves. A. A series of responses produced by increasing concentrations of agonist. B. Responses plotted as a function of the concentrations of agonist. C. General regions of dose-response curves.*

the relationship between the quantity of a substance (drug or ligand) and the graded effect that substance has on a biologic system. Historically, it is derived from studies on whole body systems, hence the term *dose* is used to describe quantity; more accurately, in vitro systems produce *concentration response curves.* A prerequisite to a discussion of dose-response curves is a consideration of dependent and independent variables.

In every experiment, there is a set of *independent variables,* the value of which does not depend on the outcome of the experiment, and a set of *dependent variables,* the value of which is determined by the experiment (Fig 2-1A). It is important to differentiate which variables are which in drug studies in order to assign significance correctly. In studies of drug action on biologic systems, the independent variables are set by the investigator and usually include drug concentration. It is assumed that only random variability is associated with independent variables. The dependent variable usually is measured from the system as biologic effect. This can take the form of either a change from a basal state or a change from a stimulated or depressed state (see Chapter 7 for further discussion). In the construction of dose-response curves, the values of the independent variable (concentration) are plotted against what is observed as the dependent variable, namely response.

Dose-response curves have three major properties: *threshold, slope,* and *maximal asymptote* (Fig 2-1B). At the least, dose-response curves should quantify system sensitivity to drugs (or, from another point of view, drug potency on a system) in an unambiguous manner. In these cases, dose-response curves may be sufficiently accurate to allow comparison of the behavior of systems to molecular models of drug action. The curves can be compared to theoretically modeled dose-response curves to gain insight into the molecular nature of the interactions.

2.1.1 Maximal Asymptote

The general shape of biologic dose-response curves, as shown in Figure 2-1B, is a threshold for effect, followed by a rapidly rising responsiveness of the system to drug concentration, followed by a decrease in the relative effect with increasing doses until no further response to increasing dose is observed. This part of the curve is the maximal asymptote. When actual concentration is used as the input axis (*x* axis), it is easy to be deceived by the initial rapidity of the responsive to dose (i.e., a steep initial curve) such that a less responsive region of the curve may mistakenly be taken to be the maximal asymptote. For example, Figure 2-2A shows a typical dose-response curve with an inferred maximal asymptote by graphic examination. However, an extension of the *x* axis (Fig 2-2B) reveals that higher doses of drug indeed would produce higher responses but our viewing window for this reaction was truncated so that this was not apparent. Such limited viewing is a common phenomenon in biology and has led to the use of *semilogarithmic* plots for dose-response curves.

Figure 2-2C shows the same dose-response curve on a semi-logarithmic scale, where the logarithm of the dose (concentration) is plotted against the response. It more clearly shows how the maximal asymptote is underestimated on a nonlogarithmic scale (compare the maximum from Fig 2-2A with the true maximum) and also allows a wider range of drug concentrations to be visualized. In general, most biologic systems respond to a 100-fold to 300-fold range of drug concentration. Such a large concentration range is difficult to accommodate on a linear scale as most of the drug effect is at the lower multiples of concentration. However, on a logarithmic scale, a 300-fold concentration range can effectively be displayed with accompanying responses. The characteristic regions of a dose-response curve on a logarithmic scale are shown in Figure 2-2D.

The most difficult parameter to estimate accurately on a dose-response curve is the maximal asymptote. This is because, theoretically, it represents the

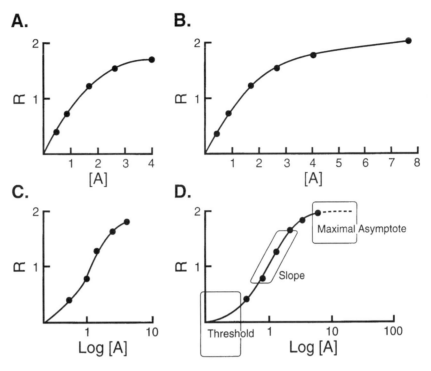

FIGURE 2-2. *Dose-response curves.* A. *Direct response plotted as a function of concentration of drug.* B. *The same curve as in A but with a twofold increase in maximal dose tested.* C. *The same curve shown in B on a semilogarithmic scale.* D. *Semilogarithmic dose-response curve showing the three major regions: threshold, slope, and maximal asymptote.*

response at infinite drug concentration, a value not possible to obtain literally but possible only to estimate. Usually, the response is measured at increasing drug concentrations until further increases in drug produce no visible increase in response. At this point, the maximal asymptote is estimated graphically.

Theoretic achievability of infinite drug concentration notwithstanding, the increase in response may be so minute as to be insignificant. Under these circumstances, a good estimate of the theoretic maximal asymptote may indeed by made. There are however, numerous conditions under which the maximal response to a drug may not easily be measured; for instance, increasing concentrations of drug may produce complicating secondary effects that obfuscate the primary response measurement. In such situations iterative computer fitting of the existing data points must suffice to estimate a maximum asymptote that otherwise is not observed (vide infra).

2.1.2 Slope

Another parameter needed to describe a dose-response curve is the slope, which dictates the pitch of the line connecting the level of response to one

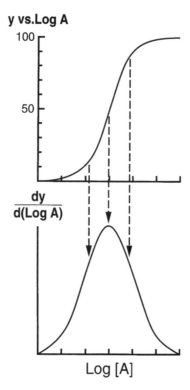

FIGURE 2-3. *Slope of a semilogarithmic dose-response curve. Bottom curve indicates the first derivative of the response (slope) as a function of the response. The slope of the curve initially increases with concentration and, at the point of half maximal response, an inflection occurs and the slope begins to decrease.*

dose to the level of response produced by another dose. The slope of dose-response curves can be somewhat linearized on a semilogarithmic scale (see Fig 2-2D). However, even when dose-response curves are represented semilogarithmically, the slope is not constant but varies with the level of response. Figure 2-3 shows the slope of a typical semi-logarithmic dose-response curve as the first derivative. It can be seen from this figure that the slope increases from the threshold to the half-maximal inflection point and then decreases again to zero. There are mathematic methods to quantify this parameter that can take this dependence on response level into consideration.

2.1.3 Dose-Response Curve Location Parameters: Potency

The measure of drug potency from a dose-response curve is the location parameter along the *x* axis. Usually, this is the concentration of drug that produces half of the maximal response referred to as the *effective dose* or the *effective concentration* for 50% maximal response (ED_{50} and EC_{50}, respectively). However, other levels of response can be used, such as ED_{30} or ED_{75} estimates (Fig 2-4).

Measures of potency usually come from semilogarithmic dose-response curves such as that shown in Figure 2-2C. Using these, the interpolated values (EC_{50}, ED_{30}, ED_{75}, etc.) are all obtained from a logarithmic scale. Given a collection of such curves yielding a collection of ED_{50} values, random variation will give a normal distribution (Fig 2-5A). It should be noted that all statistical manipulations, comparisons, and representations require a normal distribution; therefore, these values must remain on a logarithmic scale. Hence, the values should be averaged as the logarithm—that is, the *geometric mean* should be used (1). If these values were converted to actual ED_{50} values, the distribution would cease to be normal (Fig 2-5B) and all parametric statistical tests would be invalid.

It is important to note that many assessments of drug activity are metameters of changes in the dependent variable to a form of the independent variable. Thus, the activity of a drug is assessed in a biologic system, a model is made of the relationship between dose and response, and then a characteristic property of the drug is inferred from that relationship. Most often this is a calculated concentration of the drug that produces a defined response: potency (Fig 2-6A). The transform used for this purpose can affect greatly the errors in the resulting potency estimate. For example, if the transform yields a steep relationship between dose and response, then errors in the dependent variable will translate into relatively smaller errors in the independent variable (Fig 2-6B). However, if this transform is not steep, then the

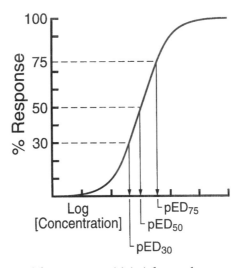

FIGURE 2-4. *Measures of drug potency (also system sensitivity) from a dose-response curve. Shown are concentrations producing 30%, 50%, and 75% maximal response. On a logarithmic scale, these values are expressed as the -log (pD value).*

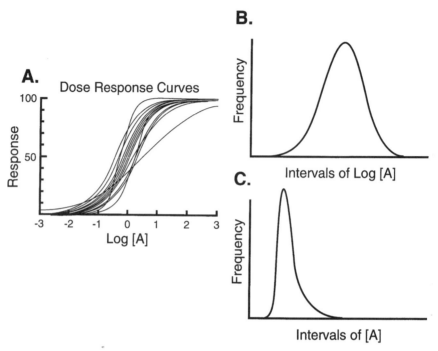

FIGURE 2-5. *Dispersion around dose-response curves. A. A sample collection of dose-response curve for a given system. B. The distribution of ED$_{50}$ values expressed as logarithms. C. The same distribution as in B but converted from logarithmic to arithmetic values. Note the skewed distribution as the very small readings approach zero. This skewed distribution cannot be used for statistical analysis.*

reverse will occur—namely, that error in the dependent variable may translate into a great deal of error in estimates of the independent variable (Fig 2-6C). This can be a factor in one's choice of test system.

Of paramount importance to this process is the fact that the accuracy of all pharmacologic estimates of drug activity relies on the accuracy of the independent variable, which is the concentration of drug at the site of biologic activity. Any errors in this estimate of concentration immediately will be transferred to the estimate of potency. This is discussed more fully in Chapter 5.

2.2 MATHEMATIC MODELING OF DOSE-RESPONSE CURVES

Usually, an array of data points is obtained experimentally, and some generalization needs to be extrapolated from their organization. An unbiased method for accomplishing this is to fit the data points mathematically to a mathematic model. A model first is chosen and then the parameters of that

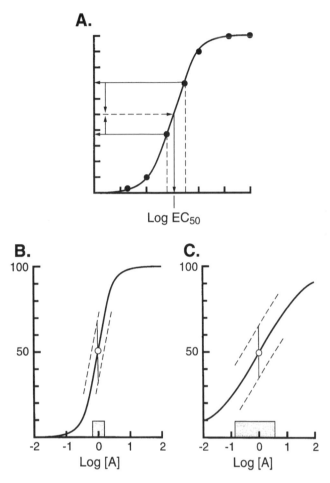

FIGURE 2-6. *Interpolation of measures of potency (in this case EC_{50}). A. Two concentrations of drug are added to the system, the response determined and, from that, the log EC_{50} interpolated (with prior knowledge of the maximal asymptote). B. A collection of steep dose-response curves yields a narrow band of EC_{50} values on the x-axis. C. In contrast, a series of shallow dose-response curves yield a wide band of EC_{50} values on the x axis.*

model are altered systematically until the deviation between the predicted data points and the actual data points is minimal.

2.2.1 Why Model Dose-Response Curves?

A dose-response curve is a representation of the behavior of a drug in a biologic system. A mathematic representation of a dose-response curve can be useful in three ways. First, it allows all the data to be used to generalize drug activity, which increases accuracy. For example, a limited dataset may yield the dose-response curve shown in Figure 2-7A. Joining the data points and estimating an ED_{50} from this curve has the inherent shortcoming of including in

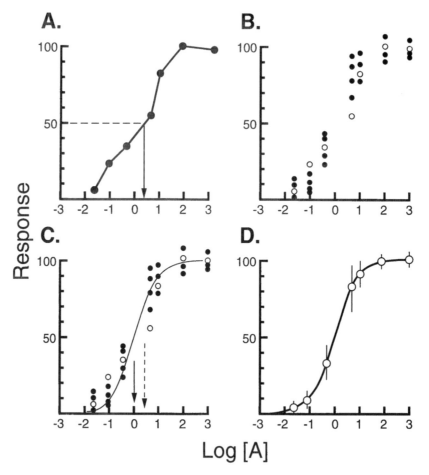

FIGURE 2-7. *Fitting of dose-response curves. A. A dose-response curve obtained by joining single esti-mates of response with straight lines. B. More estimates from the same preparation. The solid responses represent additional estimates, the open circles the original sample shown in A. C. A fit of the logistic function to the complete dataset. Note the difference in the EC_{50} value from the complete dataset (as compared to the single estimate in A). D. Data points shown as the mean response (with standard error of the means) for each concen-tration of drug.*

the estimation what may be an aberrant response (i.e., the response to a given agonist concentration may skew the result). This is attributed to a sampling error (see Chapter 9), whereby the sample chosen from the population is not representative of the entire population. It would be supposed that if this dose-response curve could be obtained an infinite number of times, the "true" dose-response curve (shown in Fig 2-7B) would be obtained along with the true ED_{50}. Curve fitting allows a general curve to be calculated from all the data points, thereby destressing the importance of the aberrant data point (Fig 2-7C) and to more closely model the true dose-response curve from a limited dataset. Under these circumstances, the ED_{50} is estimated from all 31 data points rather than from the two points joining the two responses containing the 50% maximal response ordinate.

A second reason that mathematic modeling of dose-response curves is useful is that biologic variance may be minimized when comparing different drugs in a given system. The problem of aberrant data points becomes more important when dealing with more than one dose-response curve. For example, Figure 2-8A depicts dose-response curves to two agonists from which a comparison of potency is to be made. It can be seen from the limited datasets, comparison of the ED_{30}, ED_{50}, and ED_{75} all yield values that depend on the level of measurement. This is due to the unevenness of the data. Therefore, no useful comparison for these two drugs can be made from the curves as shown. However, if dose-response curves of common slope are fit to these curves, then all the data can be used to calculate the best representation of parallel dose-response curves for these agonists (Fig 2-8B). Under these circumstances, an unbiased estimate of the relative potency can be obtained.

A third reason to model dose-response curves is that a mathematic fit of a dataset may be a useful means for comparing data to a molecular model. Before considering this idea, it is useful to discuss the type of models used in these processes. The first step is to choose a mathematic function that yields

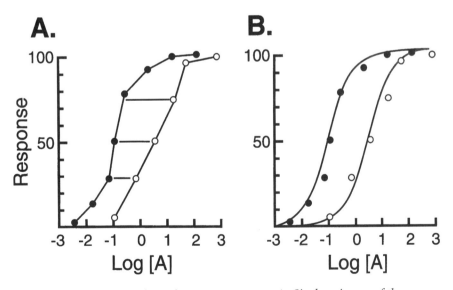

FIGURE 2-8. *The dextral displacement of two dose-response curves. A. Single estimates of the response are joined by straight lines. The magnitude of the shift to the right of the dose-response curve varies with the level of response chosen (low doses show a smaller shift than higher doses). B. Smooth logistic curves are fit to the two dose-response curves (common slope), eliminating the dose dependence of the shift measurement.*

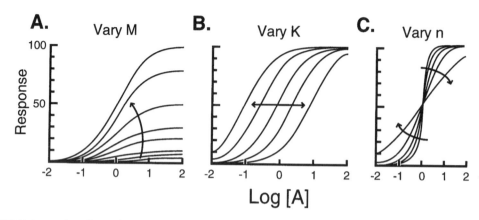

FIGURE 2-9. *The effects of varying three parameters of the logistic function on the resulting dose-response curve. A. Varying the maximum dose (M) does not change the location parameter along the x axis. B. Varying the location parameter (K) produces parallel shifts along the concentration axis. C. Varying the slope (n) changes the pitch of the dose-response curve but does not change the location along the x-axis or the maximum.*

a line with a shape similar to the array of data points, thereby increasing the likelihood of a close fit between the dose-response curve and the data points.

2.2.2 Choice of Models

One of the most useful mathematic models to fit dose-response curves is the *general logistic function* (2). Because it has both the general shape of most dose-response curves and a great deal of flexibility:

$$E = \frac{a^n M}{a^n + K^n} \qquad [2.1]$$

where E is the dependent variable, a is the value of the independent variable, M is the magnitude of the maximal asymptote, n is the slope parameter, and K is the location parameter along the independent variable axis. Figure 2-9A shows the effects of varying M (n and K constant), Figure 2-9B the effects of varying K (n and M constant), and Figure 2-9C the effects of varying n (K and M constant). With the three parameters n, M, and K, a wide variety of dose-response curves can be fit and modeled. The next step is to fit the data points iteratively to the equation for the model, which is done by nonlinear curve-fitting procedures.

2.2.3 Nonlinear Curve Fitting

The sequence employed for nonlinear curve fitting is shown in Figure 2-10. As an example, Figure 2-11A shows an array of ordinate values obtained experimentally from a set of independent variables, in this case a series of

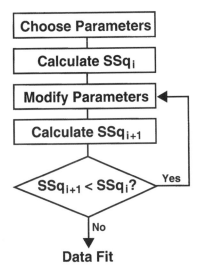

FIGURE 2-10. *Schematic of the conceptual process of fitting by the method of least sum of squares. The curve is calculated to a chosen model with an initial set of parameters. The square of the differences between the actual ordinate values and those calculated by this model is summed (to form the reference SSq). The parameters then are altered and the SSq recalculated and compared to the previous SSq. If the second SSq is smaller (closer fit to the data points), the second set of parameters is chosen as the reference set and the process is repeated. When no further diminution of the SSq can be observed, the parameters are considered optimal for that particular model.*

cellular responses to a collection of agonist concentrations. The model to be fit is the simple logistic function ($n=1$) according to the following equation:

$$y = \frac{[A]M}{[A] + K_A} \qquad [2.2]$$

where M is the maximal ordinate asymptote, and K_A is the location parameter of the dose-response curve along the x axis. Note that at this point, no molecular significance is given to the parameters; this follows the assessment of how well the data points fit to the mathematic model. The first step is to make estimates for the parameters M and K_A. For the data shown in Figure 2-11B, the first estimates will be $M = 125$ and $K_A = 5$. At this point, y values are calculated for the various values for x according to Equation 2-2, with the first estimate values for M and K_A. The difference between the calculated values for y denoted as y and actual values is then calculated. To increase the sensitivity of this difference and also to negate the sign, it is squared. The sum of squares [$SSq = \Sigma (y - y_c)^2$, where y_c refers to the calculated value and y the experimentally derived value] then becomes a measure of how well the model fits the data (i.e., if the sum of squares is large, then the fit is not optimal and,

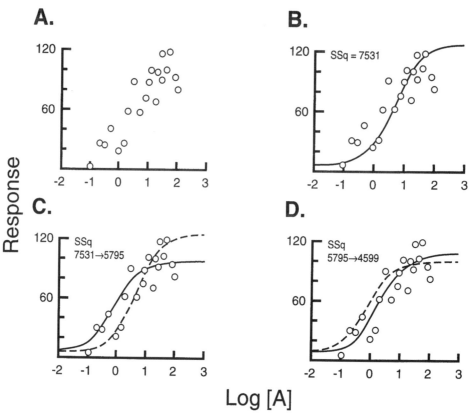

FIGURE 2-11. *Least-squares fitting of the logistic function to a dataset. A. Dose-response data points. B. The initial (reference) fit. C. Second fit. The SSq is reduced from 7531 to 5795. D. The third fit reduces the SSq from 5795 to 4599. Subsequent alteration of the parameters failed to reduce this SSq, thus the solid curve shown is the best-fit logistic curve for the data points.*

either the model is inadequate, or the estimates of the parameters are inaccurate). Therefore, the next step is to alter systematically the parameters M and K_A and recalculate SSq. This is done iteratively until no further changes in SSq result from changes in M and K_A. Figures 2-11B through 2-11D show the repeated process for the data points. At this point, the minimum least squares for the errors between the calculated and actual data points is achieved, and no further manipulation of the equation can make the model fit more closely. Then an assessment is made as to the applicability of the model to the data (see Fig 2-10). This process is accomplished readily by computer utilization of nontransformed data.

A special consideration may be required for the estimation, by curve fitting, of the maximal asymptote. As noted previously, data points often are difficult to obtain at high drug concentrations, because other secondary drug activities may obscure the true response. Under these circumstances, non-linear curve-fitting techniques may be required to estimate the maximum unobtainable experimentally. In general, the computer models will use the existing data points to best-fit the mathematic model and then will impose the maximum resulting from that fit.

There are certain mathematic transforms that apparently illuminate the maxima of dose-response curves, but these should be viewed with caution. For example, the Scatchard transformation of Equation 2.2 yields the following:

$$\frac{y}{[A]} = \frac{y}{K_A} + \frac{M}{K_A} \qquad [2.3]$$

Under these circumstances, a plot of y/x on y yields a straight line of which the x intercept is the maximum M. Figure 2-12A shows a dose-response curve and Fig 2-12B the Scatchard transformation of it. However, this transform, as

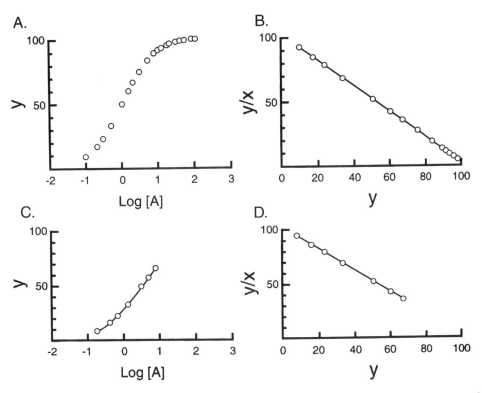

FIGURE 2-12. *Transformations of dose-response data. A. A full dose-response curve. B. Scatchard transformation (Equation 2.3) of the same data. C. A partial sample of the data points. The maximal response cannot be inferred from this curve. D. Scatchard transformation of the data shown in C. Though extrapolation of the maximal response appears to be possible, visualization of the nontransformed data in C indicates the fallacy of doing so.*

well as yielding a skewed array of errors also can yield a false sense of security with respect to the attainment of the true maximum. Figure 2-12C shows a partial dose-response curve and Fig 2-12D the Scatchard transformation of this partial dataset. Although the Scatchard plot indicates that a straight line with maximum M intercept has been achieved, the true untransformed dose-response curve (Fig 2-12C) clearly indicates that this is not true. The true maximum and the Scatchard maximum are considerably different (see Fig 2-12C).

The key to an accurate estimate of the maximum is to have as much data near the maximum as is possible. As seen in Figure 2-13A, the estimated maximum from a subset of the data that is below the true maximal response is considerably different from the maximum from a larger subset, which itself is still different from the complete dataset. In general, it is desirable to obtain data points beyond the point of inflection of the slope of the dose-response curve. This is illustrated by Figure 2-13B, which depicts the slope of the dose-response curve shown in Figure 2-13A (the first derivative of the general

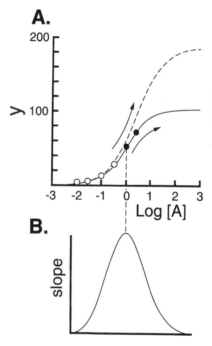

FIGURE 2-13. *The effect of the range of ordinate values on the estimation of the maximal asymptote. Two fits of the data points. The open circles (smaller sample of data) lead to an overestimation of the maximum response. The data points are all below the inflection point of the slope of the curve (bottom curve). By adding two more estimates (one of which is beyond the inflection point of the slope), a lower (and more realistic) estimate of the maximum is obtained.*

logistic function). An increase in accuracy is seen once the data points enter the region where the slope of the dose-response curve begins to decrease.

2.2.4 Comparison of Data to Models

There are mathematic models for datasets that can be derived from molecular models of drug-receptor interaction. The most simple, and best-known, of these is the Langmuir adsorption isotherm for the binding of molecules. Published in 1916 by the chemist Nobel Laureate Irving Langmuir, it is a simple formulation of the adsorption of gas molecules onto a surface (3). Thus the system can be visualized in the schematic shown in Figure 2-14 where the gas molecules (denoted by μ, using Langmuir's original formulation) either are in the unbound free gas phase or are bound to a miniscule region of the surface shown by the cross-hatched area. It is assumed that if a molecule is bound to a given area, then the binding of another molecule to the same area is precluded. The total fractional area of the surface bound by

Langmuir Adsorption Isotherm

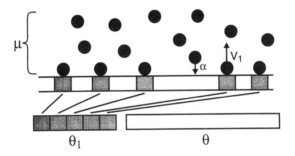

$$\text{Rate of condensation} = \alpha\theta\mu$$
$$\text{Rate of evaporation} = V_1\theta_1$$
$$\text{At equilibrium, } \alpha\theta\mu = V_1\theta_1$$
$$\theta_1 + \theta = 1$$
$$\longrightarrow \theta_1 = \frac{\alpha\mu}{\alpha\mu + V_1}$$
$$\longrightarrow \frac{\mu}{\mu + \dfrac{V_1}{\alpha}} = \frac{[A]}{[A] + K_A}$$

FIGURE 2-14. *Schematic of Langmuir's derivation of the adsorption isotherm. The bound surface (darkened area) expressed as a fraction of the total area (darkened plus white) can be calculated by a simple transform of the concentration and the equilibrium dissociation constant. The form of the equation is a special case of the general logistic function and yields sigmoidal curves.*

molecules is denoted by θ_1 whereas the remaining area is denoted as θ. The total area is given as unity, where $1 = \theta_1 + \theta$. The rate of condensation of the gas onto the surface is given by the first-order reaction rate—namely, the product of the intrinsic rate of onset (α) and the concentration of unbound molecules driving the binding reaction, which is given, in turn, by the product of the concentration of molecules (μ) and the available free area for binding (θ). The rate of evaporation of the molecules from the surface is the product of the intrinsic rate of offset from the surface (v_1) and the fraction of molecules bound (given by the product of the concentration μ and the fraction of surface already bound [θ_1]). Under equilibrium conditions, the rate of condensation will equal the rate of evaporation, thus:

$$\alpha \, \theta \, \mu = v_1 \theta_1 \qquad\qquad [2.4]$$

Substituting $1 - \theta$ for θ_1, this equation can be rearranged to the familiar Langmuir adsorption isotherm:

$$\theta_1 = \frac{\mu}{\mu + v_1/\alpha} \qquad\qquad [2.5]$$

In pharmacologic terms, this refers to ρ (the fraction of drug receptors bound by drug) in the following equation:

$$\rho = \frac{[A]}{[A] + K_A} \qquad\qquad [2.6]$$

where $[A]$ is the molar concentration of drug in the receptor compartment and K_A is the equilibrium dissociation of the drug-receptor complex. Note the similarity between this equation and Equation 1.3 derived from first principles.

Though the shape of the dose-response curve must be consistent with a molecular mechanism, it cannot be considered proof of mechanism. For example, the data points shown in Figure 2-15A that are fit by the Langmuir adsorption isotherm also can be fit by other equations. As seen in Figure 2-15B, $y = M*(1 - e^{-kx})$ also yields an apparently good fit of the data points, thereby producing a conundrum. The method of *normalization of residuals* sometimes may be used to determine which model is more appropriate. Specifically, the sum of the squares should represent only random error and should not be related to the magnitude of the independent variable. However, if the pattern of the residuals, as plotted with values of x, is not randomly distributed, then a systematic error is suggested, which, in turn, suggests that the model chosen to fit the data is inappropriate. For example, the two equations used to fit the data points in Figure 2-15A and B appear, by eye, to be equivalent. However, Figure 2-15B shows the residuals [$\Sigma \, (y - y_c)^2$ val-

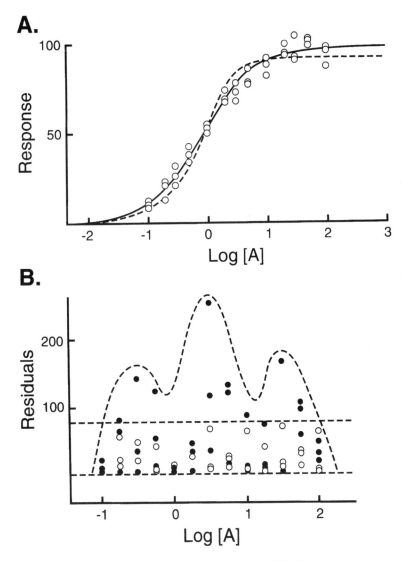

FIGURE 2-15. *Distribution of residuals as an aid to choosing fitting models for dose-response curves. A. Data points fit to two models, the logistic (solid line) and an exponential (dotted line). B. The residuals (differences between calculated and actual values) for the logistic fit are distributed evenly along the concentration axis (indicating a balanced fit; open circles). In contrast, the exponential yields residuals with extreme values in selected regions of the concentration range (solid circles). This unbalanced spectrum of residuals indicates that the exponential model is not as good a model for the data points.*

Total Drug Activity

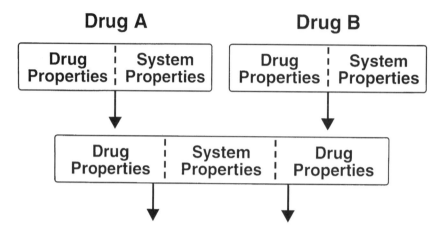

FIGURE 2-16. *Schematic of the concept of the null method. Drug effect is an amalgam of expression of drug properties translated by the biologic system. Measurement of the effects of two drugs in the same tissue system allows cancellation of the system translation effects of drug properties and, therefore, comparison of only drug properties.*

ues] and how the Langmuir isotherm provides a random scatter of residuals as opposed to the exponential function $y = M*(1-e^{-kx})$. The analysis of residuals provides added information in the choice of model used to fit data (see Fig 2-10).

2.3 NULL METHODS

Biologic systems are extremely complex. Moreover, when they are manipulated in experiments, it generally is not known to what extent the biologic system is altered. The major approach used to cancel the impact of such complexity is the *null method*, the major tenet of which is that *a single change is made in an otherwise common field*. The null method is most effective when minimal changes (or, if possible, a single change) are made.

The null method is most evident in the comparison of dose-response curves to various agonists or a single agonist in systems in which other factors relating to the receptor have been altered (i.e., receptor antagonism). Figure 2-16 is a schematic representation of the power of the null method. The activity of an agonist is a result of a number of receptor-related drug properties as well as the way in which the biologic system translates those properties (see Fig 1-3). The key feature of the null method is that equal biologic system responses to a drug are considered to activate equally the biologic system determinants of response. Therefore, comparison of so-called equiactive responses negates the translation effects of the system and compares only the drug specific properties that determine response. This is the single most important tool in pharmacology because it allows drugs to be compared with one another and does not link activity with the type of biologic system, which is critical in the estimation of properties such as efficacy. Unlike affinity, where a chemical constant can be assigned, efficacy has no absolute scale. Therefore, the major method of denoting the strength of one drug's ability to produce a response is to compare it to another; for example, drug A has 10 times the intrinsic efficacy of drug B.

2.4 SYNOPSIS

This chapter presents the following ideas:

- Experimental data are ordered in terms of independent variables (those set by the experimenter and assumed to be known, such as drug concentration added to the system) and dependent variables (those observed and resulting from interaction of the drug with the system).

- Dose-response curves present dependent variables as a function of independent variables. They have three basic features—namely, threshold, slope, and maximal asymptote.

- The maximal asymptote is difficult to estimate experimentally but is best visualized in semi-logarithmic dose-response curves.

- The location parameter of a dose-response curve quantifies the potency of the drug (and the sensitivity of the system to the drug). Because they are estimated from a semilogarithmic curve, drug potencies should be expressed as geometric means.

- The influence of errant data points is reduced and better accuracy results when dose-response curves are fit to mathematic models.

- A very flexible model for dose-response curves is the general logistic function. Minimization of sum-of-squares calculations can be used to obtain the best fit of data points to a calculated curve.

- The most useful first model to compare drug-binding data is the Langmuir adsorption isotherm for binding to homogeneous noninteracting sites. Patterns of residuals can assist in determining the correct model for fitting curves.

■ The most powerful method for delineating drug effects from system effects is the null method.

REFERENCES

1. Fleming WW, Westfall DP, De La Lande IS, Jellet LB. Log-normal distribution of equieffective doses of norepinephrine and acetylcholine in several tissues. J Pharmacol Exp Ther 1972;181:339–345.
2. Waud DR. Analysis of dose-response relationships. In: Narahashi TL, Bianchi CP, eds. Advances in general and cellular pharmacology. New York: Plenum, 1976: 145–178.
3. Langmuir I. The constitution and fundamantal properties of solids and liquids. J Am Chem Soc 1916; 38: 2221–2229.

FURTHER READING

Dowd JE, Riggs DS. A comparison of estimates of Michaelis-Menten kinetic constants from various linear transformations. J Biol Chem 1965;240:863-869.

Gaddum JH. Bioassays and mathematics. Pharmacol Rev 1953;5:87–134.

Motulsky HJ, Rasnas LA. Fitting curves to data using non-linear regression: A practical and nonmathematical view. 1987;1:365–374.

Plumbridge TW, Aarons LJ, Brown JR. Problems associated with analysis and interpretation of small molecule/macromolecule binding data. 1978;30:69–74.

Riggs DS. The mathematical approach to physiological problems. Baltimore:Williams and Wilkins, 1963.

Tallarida RJ, Murray RG. Manual of pharmacologic calculations with computer programs. Berlin: Springer-Verlag, 1979.

Molecular Models of Drug-Receptor Interaction

IN THIS CHAPTER, the origins of the mathematic descriptions of drug-receptor interaction are discussed. Specifically derived from mass action kinetics at the turn of the century, equations by A J Clark formed the framework of receptor theory (section 3.1). The ability of drugs to produce physiologic response was described by theoretic constants introduced by Ariens and, later, by Stephenson. The resulting equations formed the basis of occupation theory. From electrophysiologic studies on ion channels came a revolutionary idea regarding receptor theory—namely, two-state theory (section 3.2). From this and the idea that receptors could form hetero-trimeric species in biologic membranes came the development of more specific mathematic models of receptor mechanisms. Section 3.3 outlines the general methods used to create mathematic models. The next section (3.4) discusses a widespread receptor motif, the ternary complex formed among drugs, receptors, and membrane bound coupling proteins. A related theoretic framework for the functional study of receptors, the operational model, is discussed in section 3.5. These ideas are reviewed in the chapter synopsis (3.6).

3.1 RECEPTOR THEORY: HISTORIC PERSPECTIVE

Throughout medical history, doctors and scientists have been intrigued by the magic of medicines whereby minute amounts of some substances produce radical changes in human behavior and health. The receptor concept was implied throughout that history. As early as 1685, Robert Boyle suggested that different parts of the body have different textures, and therefore, different bound substances; a rudimentary idea suggesting the existence of drug receptors.

The concept of receptors is credited to two eminent physiologists, John Newport Langley and Paul Ehrlich. Central to their independent studies was the concept of the dependence of physiologic action on chemical structure. While a student at Cambridge in 1874, Langley explained the antagonism of pilocarpine by atropine. In a paper published in 1878, he foreshadowed the receptor concept: "...There is a substance or substances in the nerve endings or gland cells with which both atropine and pilocarpine are capable of forming compounds."

In that same year, Paul Ehrlich graduated from the University of Leipzig and, in his thesis on histologic staining, suggested that staining was the result of a chemical interaction between two compounds. His later work on immunization discussed "receptive side chains." Ehrlich, having read the work of Emil Fischer who formulated a theory of enzyme action, suggested that these side chains interacted with toxins as a lock and key. These ideas guided his later great work in the field of chemotherapy.

It was a student at Cambridge University, A J Clark , who first applied mathematic principles to drug receptor theory. He studied the effects of acetylcholine on various isolated tissues and noted that the relationship between drug concentration and response corresponded closely to the equation (1):

$$K \cdot x = y/(100 - y) \tag{3.1}$$

where x is the drug concentration and y is the percentage of the maximal response to the drug. A rearrangement of Equation 3.1 shows the form of the familiar Langmuir adsorption isotherm:

$$y = \frac{100\,x}{x + 1/K} \tag{3.2}$$

Clark published a treatise in 1937 that summarized and extended the existing theories of drug-receptor interaction. The major problem at this time was the lack of knowledge about the relationship between receptor occupancy and tissue response. Therefore, the simplest assumptions were made in Clark's treatise:

- The maximal response to a drug (E_m) was the tissue maximal response.

- Fractional tissue response (E_A/E_m) was directly equal to fractional receptor occupancy ($[A \cdot R]/[R_t]$).

Under these circumstances, the following equation represents the response of a drug A in a tissue, as described by Clark:

$$\frac{E_A}{E_m} = \frac{[A \cdot R]}{[R_t]} = \frac{[A]}{[A] + K_A} \qquad [3.3]$$

where K_A is the equilibrium dissociation constant of the drug-receptor complex. Clark recognized that the relationship between receptor occupation by a drug and the resulting response was not a linear one in most cases and that therefore drug effect, as described by Equation 3.3, was limited.

The impact of Langley's and Ehrlich's and, even later, of Clark's, ideas was limited in their lifetimes because they involved molecular concepts in a technology that could not experimentally test them. This was to change with the concept of bioassay. Although a diverse number of scientific disciplines contributed to the concept of specific receptors for chemicals in biologic systems, it was through the method of bioassay that the critical data for the formulation of receptor theory were obtained. Bioassay, the quantitative measurement of drug effect in intact biologic systems, was pioneered by the great pharmacologists Sir John Gaddum, Sir Henry Dale, and Harold Burn (2).

The first prerequisite of bioassay was that the measuring system be stable. The state of the art in pharmacology into the first half of the twentieth century consisted of a great deal of anecdotal knowledge and creative expertise in sustaining whole biologic preparations over periods of time during which changes in tissue state were measured with drug challenge. The major tool for quantitative pharmacology was the isolated tissue. Thus, whole organs were placed in heated chambers and incubated with physiologic salt solutions, kept at physiologic pH, and perfused with oxygen such that they behaved as in the intact organism. The difference was that the volume perfusing the preparation (and therefore the receptors) was known, and thus the concentration of drugs at the receptors also was known (with the obvious caveats to this assumption discussed in Chapter 5).

A typical isolated tissue system is shown in Figure 3-1. The tissue is placed in a heated organ bath, and organ function (i.e., contraction) is recorded on a simple apparatus called a *kymograph* which consists of a lever, one end of which is tied to the tissue and the other to a pen that presses on a smoked rotating drum by gravity. As the tissue contracts, either spontaneously or in response to a drug, the lever is pulled upward and a record of the displace-

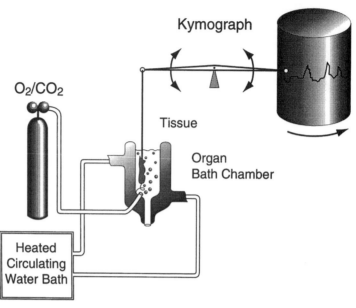

FIGURE 3-1. *Schematic diagram depicting an organ bath life support system for an isolated tissue. The tissue is bathed in heated physiologic fluid containing nutrients and oxygen at the required pH. Contractions and relaxations of the tissue are recorded via a string attached to a lever which, when displaced, creates a record on a smoked revolving drum (kymograph).*

ment is scratched on the film of smoke. Bioassay enabled pharmacologists to study the effects of changing chemical structure of biologic activity. This led to the reconstruction of receptor theory to accommodate the behavior of drugs on receptors. With the quantification of drug effect using bioassay, pharmacologists began a dialogue with medicinal chemists to improve the activity of known biologically active substances, and the science of drug discovery was born. Figure 3-2 shows an early structure activity relationship for a series of catecholamines on tracheal muscle relaxation for eventual use in asthma therapy (3).

At this time, the stage was set to explore the interaction of drugs and receptors in greater depth. Relatively accurate measurements of drug response could be made and the results compared to the theory set forth by Clark. The first casualty of this scrutiny was the assumption that the tissue response was directly proportional to the drug concentration. To account for the discrepancy, a proportionality factor was introduced by E J Ariens. This constant was used to account for the fact that some agonists produced maximal responses that were less than the maximal responses to other agonists. He termed this proportionality constant *intrinsic activity* (denoted α); insertion of this term gave the effect of a drug as (4):

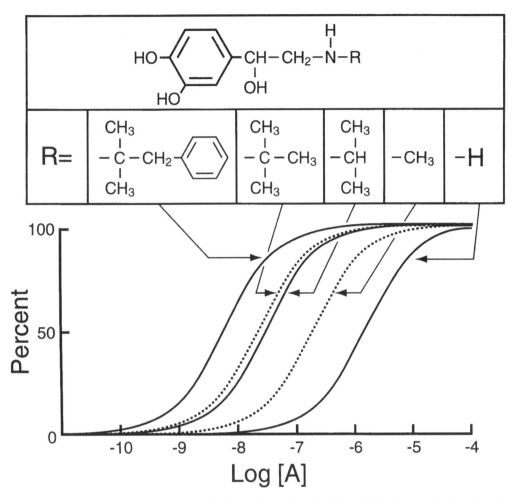

FIGURE 3-2. *Structure activity relationship for a chemical series of catecholamines producing relaxation of rat isolated trachea. It can be seen from this figure that different R substituents on the amino function produce increasing bronchodilation.*

$$\frac{E_A}{E_m} = \frac{[A \cdot R]}{[R_t]} = \frac{\alpha[A]}{[A] + K_A} \qquad [3.4]$$

The scale for α was unity for full agonists to 0 for antagonists that produced no direct tissue response. A value for α of 0.4 meant that the agonist could produce 40% of the tissue maximal response (partial agonist). Though this went a long way toward making the models of drug effect more closely align with experimental results, there still was no provision for the observation that some agonists produced maximal responses at considerably lower relative values of receptor occupancy (i.e., a 90% maximal response could be achieved for drugs when they apparently occupied only 5% to 10% of the receptors). A British pharmacologist, R P Stephenson proposed another theoretic concept to account for this disparity. He introduced the term *stimulus* and proposed that drugs produced a stimulus according to the following equation (5):

$$S = \frac{e[A]}{[A] + K_A}$$ [3.5]

where *e* was a proportionality constant called *efficacy*. The strength of this approach was that tissue response, the experimentally observed parameter, was considered some monotonic function of stimulus:

$$\frac{E_A}{E_m} = f(S) = f\left[\frac{e[A]}{[A] + K_A}\right]$$ [3.6]

The monotonic function was given the name the *stimulus-response relationship*. This was an extremely important advance in receptor pharmacology as it allowed for receptor events (activation of the receptor) to be separated from the tissue event of physiologic activity. This, in turn, allowed for receptor drug and receptor properties to be isolated from the biologic system and for statements to be made that transcended the tissue from which the data were obtained. As shown in Figure 3-3, the receptor occupancy of a drug defined

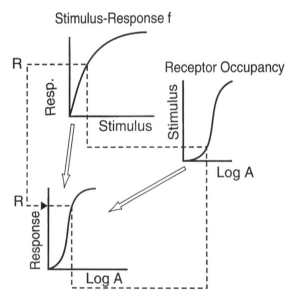

FIGURE 3-3. *The relationship between receptor occupancy and tissue response as defined by Stephenson. A given receptor occupancy by an agonist produces a given amount of stimulus which, in turn, feeds into the stimulus-response function inherent in the tissue to produce a given magnitude of response.*

the abscissal axis of the stimulus-response relationship, and this secondary process controlled the amount of tissue response obtained from a given level of occupancy. The separation of the binding of a drug to the receptor population and the resulting physiological response allowed for a number of conceptual advances in receptor theory.

3.2 TWO-STATE THEORY

Two major ideas revolutionized receptor theory in the years after Stephenson presented efficacy and stimulus. The first of these came from studies on ion channels. In general, the study of the interaction of drugs with different conformations of the same protein was hampered by adequate assay methods to differentiate the respective complexes between the drug and the different conformations. However, this became possible for certain ion channels because one of the conformations was an open ion channel that allowed the flow of ions and another was a closed ion channel. Therefore, here was an assay system that could differentiate the two protein states.

Different drugs were found to promote the flow of ions through channels, and subsequent work showed that this was because the drugs preferentially bound to the open state of the ion channel. This finding formed the basis for two-state theory. The equilibria between the two receptor states R_i and R_a and the binding of the ligand A are shown as follows (6):

$$
\begin{array}{ccc}
 & L & \\
R_i & \rightleftharpoons & R_a \\
\updownarrow K & & \updownarrow \alpha K \\
A & & A
\end{array}
\qquad [3.7]
$$

The constant describing the relative existing proportions of R_i and R_a is given by L, termed the *allosteric constant* (i.e., $L = [R_a]/[R_i]$). The equilibrium association constant of the R_i form of the receptor and the ligand is denoted as K, and for the R_a form of the receptor and ligand A as αK. Thus, the differential factor for the difference in the affinity of A for the two receptor forms is given by α (Fig 3-4). Unless a ligand has identical affinities for the two protein conformations, it preferentially binds to one of them, and this preferential binding removes that conformation from the dynamic equilibrium between the two forms and shifts it toward that particular form.

Two-state theory is important to the understanding of receptor function, as it offers a molecular and chemical mechanism for a drug actively changing a dynamic physiologic system. Thus, simply by having differential affinity for two pre-existing protein conformations, a drug can shift the relative proportions of these proteins in the system. This idea will be developed further in discussions on agonist efficacy (see Chapter 6).

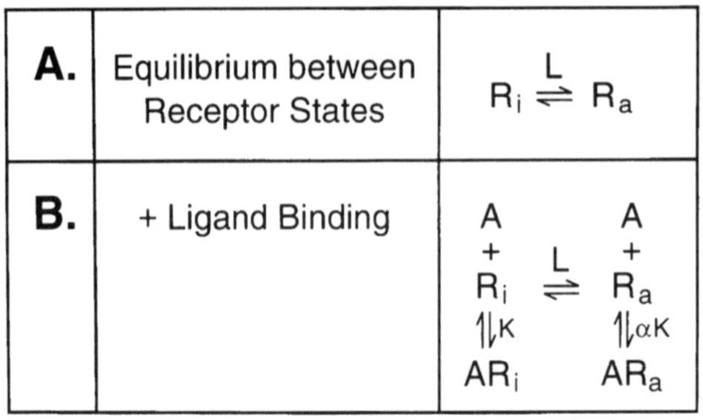

A.	Equilibrium between Receptor States	$R_i \overset{L}{\rightleftharpoons} R_a$
B.	+ Ligand Binding	$\begin{array}{ccc} A & & A \\ + & & + \\ R_i & \overset{L}{\rightleftharpoons} & R_a \\ \updownarrow K & & \updownarrow \alpha K \\ AR_i & & AR_a \end{array}$

FIGURE 3-4. *Two-state receptor theory.* A. *Schematic diagram depicting a receptor in two conformational states, active (R_a) and inactive (R_i), with respect to interaction with other membrane proteins.* B. *The interaction of a drug A in a two-state receptor system. The affinity of A for the inactive state is K. The affinity for the active state is modified by a factor α.*

The second major idea to revolutionize receptor theory was that some receptors on the cell membrane translocate in the two-dimensional space of the membrane and interact with other membrane-bound proteins to initiate physiologic function. This idea, first proposed by Pedro Cuatrecasas, led to the description of heterotrimeric models of drug action consisting of drugs, receptors, and membrane-bound coupling proteins that associated to different degrees on binding of drug (7). In general, there are numerous receptor systems that consist of a receptor for chemical ligands (recognition and transduction unit) existing in (at least) two states and that interact differentially (depending on which of the two states predominates) with other membrane-bound proteins. This type of system (heterotrimeric complexes of ligand-receptor coupler) is a recurring motif in receptor biology. The most prevalent type of heterotrimeric system is the seven-transmembrane receptor (*7TM*). This receptor resides on the cell membrane and is one of the main, if not *the* main, type of information portal for cells and extracellular chemicals. The current model for seven-transmembrane receptors, termed the *ternary complex model* (8), outlines a dynamic equilibrium between receptors and membrane-bound proteins called G-proteins, which go on to activate various effectors in cells. These G-proteins are themselves heterotrimeric proteins that have an intrinsic enzyme activity for the degradation of guanosine triphosphate and that also dissociate upon activation by receptor. The dissociated subunits migrate to effectors such as the enzyme adenylate cyclase or various ion channels to induce cellular response. It is postulated that physiologic response emanates from a receptor-activated G-protein, either R_aG or $A \cdot R_aG$. This latter species is a ternary complex among receptor, drug, and G-protein—hence the name *ternary complex model.*

The concept of a ternary complex can be generalized to the formation of *receptor heterotrimers,* consisting of a drug, a receptor, and another protein of origin specific to the receptor. Thus for seven-transmembrane receptors, the other protein is a G-protein; for one-transmembrane receptors the other protein could be another identical receptor (receptor homodimers) or another subunit of the receptor (receptor heterodimers) or an accessory protein. For nuclear proteins, the other species could be DNA. In all cases, the idea of a ternary species greatly facilitates the selectivity with which a cell can choose incoming signals and also acts as a good method of amplification. These ideas are developed more fully in Chapter 6.

3.3 MATHEMATIC MODELS OF RECEPTOR SYSTEMS

3.3.1 Common Themes

A great deal of insight into the behavior of complex systems, that otherwise would not be intuitively obvious, can be gained by building a mathematic model. There are certain common themes to these models that can be used for simple and complex systems. For example, the simple ternary complex model for 7TM receptors can be shown as: $A \cdot R$

$$[A] + [R] \xrightarrow{K_1} [A \cdot R] + [G] \xrightarrow{K_2} [A \cdot R \cdot G] \tag{3.8}$$

The first step is to derive the expressions for the equilibrium constants. This usually is done for association constants, which are defined as the quotient of the end products of the reactions divided by the reactants. Thus:

$$K_1 = \frac{[A \cdot R]}{[A][R]} \ and \ K_2 = \frac{[A \cdot R \cdot G]}{[A \cdot R][G]} \tag{3.9}$$

Then, the conservation equation for the common reactant—in this case the receptor—is stated. For this system, the total receptor concentration ($[R]_{total}$) is distributed between the receptor bound by ligand ($[A \cdot R]$), the receptor in the form of the ternary complex ($[A \cdot R \cdot G]$), and the remaining free unbound receptor ($[R]$):

$$[R]_{total} = [R] + [A \cdot R] + [A \cdot R \cdot G] \tag{3.10}$$

Thus, to derive an equation for a ratio of species of interest, both of those species must be expressed in terms of a common member of the conservation equation to allow cancellation. For example, a useful ratio for the preceding system would be the amount of ternary complex ($[A \cdot R \cdot G]$) produced by drug A as a fraction of the total receptor number ($[R]_{total}$). This would approximate the response to drug A if the ternary complex were a response-producing element. Because the ratio needed is $[A \cdot R \cdot G]/[R]_{total}$, $[R]_{total}$ needs to be expressed all in terms of $[A \cdot R \cdot G]$ to allow cancellation of the $[A \cdot R \cdot G]$ term.

From the equations describing K_1 and K_2, the following rearrangements can be made to express $[A \cdot R]$ and $[R]$ in terms of $[A \cdot R \cdot G]$ exclusively:

$$[A \cdot R] = \frac{[A \cdot R \cdot G]}{K_2[G]} \text{ and } [R] = \frac{[A \cdot R \cdot G]}{K_1 K_2[G]} \qquad [3.11]$$

Substituting for $[A \cdot R]$ and $[R]$ in the conservation equation yields:

$$[R]_{total} = [A \cdot R \cdot G](1 + 1/K_2[G] + 1/[A]K_1[G]K_2) \qquad [3.12]$$

This makes the ratio of ternary complex produced by drug to total receptor concentration ($[A \cdot R \cdot G]/[R]$):

$$\frac{[A \cdot R \cdot G]}{[R]} = \frac{[A \cdot R \cdot G]}{[A \cdot R \cdot G](1 + (1/[G]K_2) + (1/([A]K_1[G]K_2))} \qquad [3.13]$$

At this point, it is useful to express the equation in terms of dissociation constants instead of association constants. The latter parameters (in this model, K_1 and K_2) are useful in the early stages of constructing the model, as the overall association constant for a multistage reaction is simply the product of the individual association constants. For example, the overall constant for a string of concatenated isomerizations of a receptor from the binding of $[A]$ to $[R]$ to the production of $A \cdot R_3$ is controlled by the association constant $K_1 K_2 K_3$:

$$[A] + [R] \xrightleftharpoons{K_1} [A \cdot R] \xrightleftharpoons{K_2} [A \cdot R_2] \xrightleftharpoons{K_3} [A \cdot R_3] \qquad [3.14]$$

However, once the equation is formulated into the terms using the concentration of drugs, it is more meaningful to convert the equilibrium constants into the reciprocal of the association constants (they then become the equilibrium dissociation constants for the drug-receptor complex), because these contain the units of concentration and can readily be equated with the drug concentrations used in the equation. For example, the reciprocal of the association constant represents the concentration of drug that half-maximally saturates the process. Thus $1/K_1$ is denoted K_A and serves as a scale for the concentration of drug producing the effect (i.e., when $[A]/K_A = 1$, then the drug is present at the receptor at a concentration that binds to half of the population of receptors). Under these circumstances:

$$\frac{[A \cdot R \cdot G]}{[R]} = \rho = \frac{[A]/K_A \, ([G]/K_G)}{[A]/K_A \, (1 + ([G]/K_G)) + 1} \qquad [3.15]$$

Figure 3-5A shows the production of the ternary complex $[A \cdot R \cdot G]$ expressed as a fraction of $[R]$ according to Equation 3.15 and the effect of different

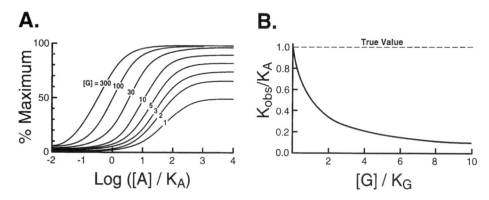

FIGURE 3-5. A. *Dose-response curves calculated according to Equation 3.15 for receptor activation by an agonist in the presence of varying concentrations of G-protein. The receptor, agonist, and G-protein form a ternary complex.* B. *The effect of the quantity of G-protein on the observed affinity of the agonist in the system (alternatively, the observed sensitivity of the system to the agonist). As the ratio of G-protein to receptor increases, so does the observed potency of the agonist.*

concentrations of $[G]$ in the receptor system. It can be seen from this figure that increases in the amount of G make the system more sensitive to the agonist.

It is worth discussing another technique in modeling—namely, the identification of equivalents. For example, the Langmuir adsorption isotherm written in the form given in Equation 3.16 has the characteristics of a maximal asymptote denoted by M and a sensitivity denoted by K_A (see Chapter 2).

$$\rho = \frac{[A]\,M}{[A] + K_A} \qquad [3.16]$$

The latter term K_A defines the location of the dose-response curve along the concentration axis and thus both the drug potency and system sensitivity. Therefore, by analogy, Equation 3.15 placed into the same general form yields a sensitivity factor (denoted K_{obs}) equal to:

$$K_{obs} = \frac{K_A}{(1 + ([G]/K_G))} \qquad [3.17]$$

This mathematic manipulation yields a meaningful physiologic relationship in that it shows that the observed sensitivity of the drug-receptor process will be greater than that controlled by the equilibrium dissociation constant of the drug-receptor complex (K_A). The greater the concentration of secondary coupling protein ($[G]$), the more driven will be the second binding process which, in turn, will pull the reaction between drug and receptor further to the right. Alternatively, the more avid the coupling process (low value for K_G), the more driven the secondary coupling will be causing enhancement of the potency of A. This was seen in the dose-response curves shown in Figure 3-5A. The effect of $[G]/K_G$ on the observed potency of A is shown in Figure 3-5B. This particular mechanism will be discussed more fully in Chapter 6.

3.3.2 Microscopic Reversibility

Another very useful concept in designing receptor models is microscopic reversibility (9). In general, this term refers to the fact that the pathways to different species must have an equal cost in terms of energy. Figure 3-6 shows a two-state receptor model in which both receptor conformations bind drug A. The equilibrium between R_i and R_a is controlled by L, and the binding of A to R_i is controlled by K. The binding of A to R_a is controlled by another constant, and it is useful to consider this to be some multiple or fraction of K, denoted αK. Specifically, if the free energy of binding of A to R_i is given by ΔF_1, and the free energy of conversion from R_i to R_a is given by ΔF_2, then two additional free energies of binding must be defined when A interacts with R_i and R_a together. Thus, an energy $\Delta F_{1,2}$ defines the free energy of A binding to receptor R_a, and an energy $\Delta F_{2,1}$ defines the free energy of conversion of R_i to R_a with drug A bound to the receptor. Under these circumstances, microscopic reversibility dictates that:

$$\Delta F_{AR_a} = \Delta F_i - \Delta F_{1,2} = \Delta F_2 - \Delta F_{2,1} \qquad [3.18]$$

The coupling factor for the influence of A on receptor interconversion (from R_i to R_a) then is given by:

$$\alpha = e^{-(\Delta F_{AR_a}/RT)} \qquad [3.19]$$

Under these circumstances, the term α sometimes comes out in factoring and clear trends can be seen in the final equation. The process from R_i to AR_a is controlled by the association constant K_{reaction} (see Fig 3-6) which, in turn, is given by αLK (see Equation 3.14 for concatenated isomerization). Though the association constant for R_i to AR_a may not be known (denoted by X in Fig 3-6), by the concept of microscopic reversibility it is fixed in that the product of the constants from R_i to AR_i and from AR_i to AR_a must have the same total association equilibrium constant as the alternative route, namely αLK. Therefore, this fixes the association rate constant for the fourth arm of the square at αL. The concept of microscopic reversibility can be extremely useful in modeling, as unknown constants, describing equilibria between species that are associated by known pathways, can be inferred.

The previous techniques then can be used to derive an equation for the

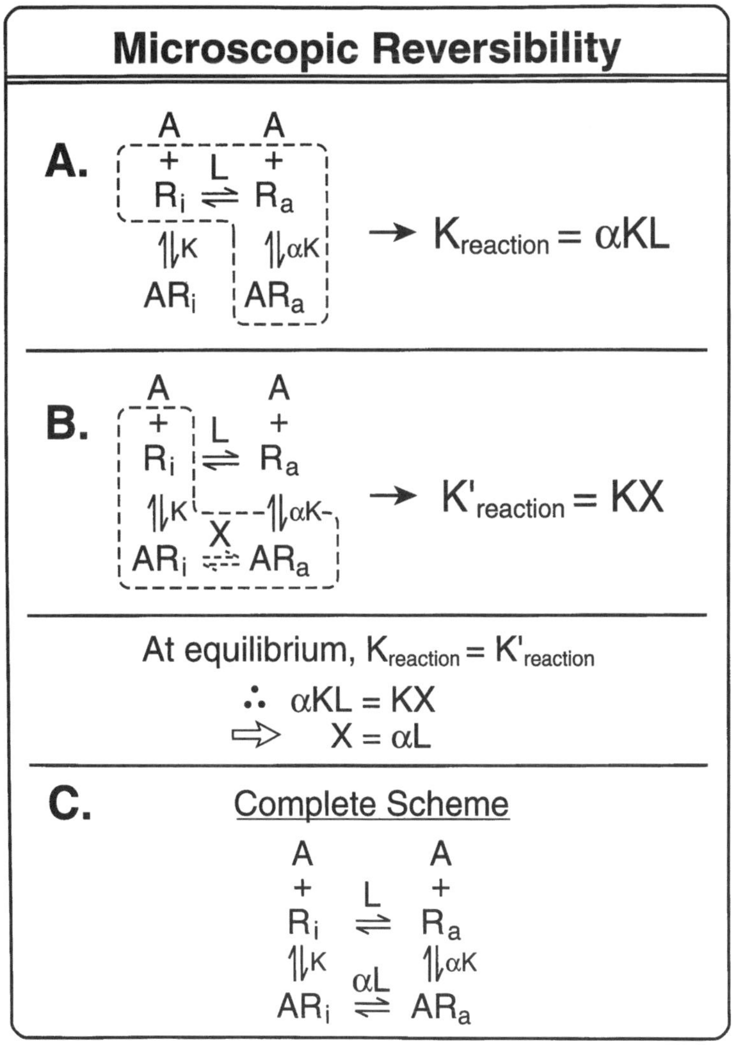

FIGURE 3-6. *The concept of microscopic reversibility. In general, this schematic demonstrates that the constants controlling the path from R_i to AR_a are equal, whether the route goes through R_a or AR_i.*

drug effects on the two-state system shown in Figure 3-4. Thus, the equilibrium equations are:

$$L = \frac{[R_a]}{[R_i]} \; and \; K = \frac{[AR_i]}{[A][R_i]} \qquad [3.20]$$

$$\alpha L = \frac{[AR_a]}{[AR_i]} \; and \; \alpha K = \frac{[AR_a]}{[A][R_a]} \qquad [3.21]$$

and the conservation equation is:

$$[R] = [R_i] + [R_a] + [AR_a] + [AR_i] \qquad [3.22]$$

The desired term for drug effect (the amount of active receptor complex produced by drug A) is $[AR_a]/[R]$ (denoted as ρ); therefore, all the terms in the conservation equation need to be converted into those containing only AR_a as the receptor species:

$$[AR_i] = \frac{[AR_a]}{\alpha K_1} \; and \; [R_a] = \frac{[AR_a]}{\alpha K [A]} \qquad [3.23]$$

$$[R_i] = \frac{[AR_i]}{[A] K} = \frac{[AR_a]}{\alpha L K [A]} \qquad [3.24]$$

Under these circumstances:

$$\rho = \frac{\alpha KL [A]}{1 + K + [A] K + \alpha KL [A]} \qquad [3.25]$$

Following the convention of converting the association constants L and K to equilibrium dissociation constants with units of concentration ($K_{act} = 1/L$ and $K_A = 1/K$):

$$\rho = \frac{[A]/K_A (\alpha/K_{act})}{[A]/K_A (1 + \alpha K_{act}) + ((1 + K_A)/K_A)} \qquad [3.26]$$

Again it can be seen that the observed apparent equilibrium constant from a dose-response curve (K_{obs}) is:

$$K_{obs} = \frac{K_A}{1 + (\alpha/K_{act})} \qquad [3.27]$$

Under these circumstances, the greater the selectivity that the drug has for the active receptor (the higher the value for α), the more potent will it be. Alternatively, the greater number of active receptors there are in the system (i.e., the smaller is K_{act} or, alternatively, the larger is L), the higher will be the potency of A.

3.4 THE TERNARY COMPLEX MODEL OF 7TM RECEPTORS

A very large class of receptors for hormones, neurotransmitters, and autacoids exists on the outside of the cell membrane and transmits information from the extracellular to the intracellular space. These receptors are structured as a succession of loops that traverse the cell membrane seven times (Fig 3-7); thus

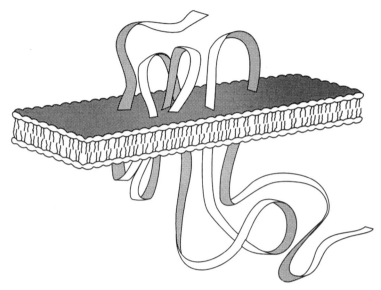

FIGURE 3-7. *Cartoon of a seven-transmembrane receptor. This major class of receptor protein functions as the cell's communications link with its environment. It consists of three extracellular and three intracellular loops of protein and seven membrane-spanning regions. Hormones and other chemicals access the receptor from the extracellular space, and the presence of these drugs is sensed by the receptor, thus transmitting a conformational change to the intracellular loops and the cytoplasm of the cell.*

they are referred to as *seven-transmembrane* or 7TM *receptors*. A pivotal model for the action of this very important class of receptor—termed the ternary complex model—was developed in 1980 by DeLean and Lefkowitz (8) and extended 12 years later by the same group. This model serves as a template for receptor models in general as it embodies two general principles common to many, namely the existence of receptors in different conformational states and the interaction of the receptor with other membrane-bound proteins by diffusion translocation. A thermodynamically complete version of the ternary complex, derived by Weiss, Morgan, and Lutz (10), is shown in Figure 3-8. This model embodies three basic interactions: the dynamic equilibrium between active and inactive receptor (face I), the interaction of the receptor with G-protein (face II) and the influence of drug binding to these two processes (face III).

The essential complexity of this model illustrates a general motif in receptor models. Specifically, models can be classified on the basis of their complexity (i.e., the number of parameters required to define the model) and also on the basis of how easily the parameters can be uniquely identified (Fig 3-9). In the lower left-hand corner of Figure 3-9 reside models of which little is known about the system (therefore the model is, by necessity, simple) and

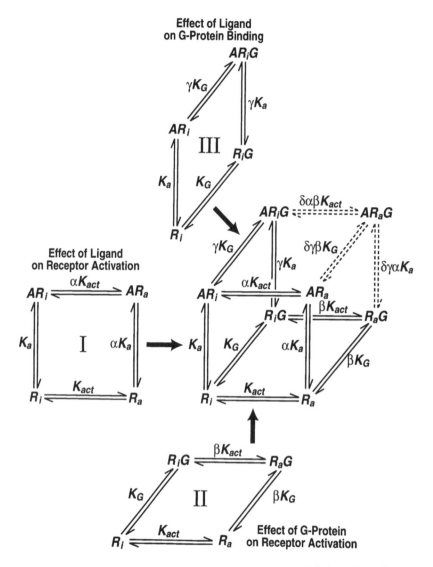

FIGURE 3-8. *A model of a seven-transmembrane receptor "system." This model shows how the receptor can exist in active ($[R_a]$) and inactive ($[R_i]$) states and how these interact with a drug designated [A] (face I). The two receptor states also can interact with membrane-bound G-proteins (face II), and the ligand can affect this interaction (face III). The result is a thermodynamic cube controlled by a number of equilibrium constants.*

little can be estimated. Such models are caricatures of biologic systems. The other extreme resides in the top right-hand corner of Figure 3-9 where a large number of parameters are required to describe the experimental situation and the parameters can be estimated independently. Under these circumstances, the model is able to simulate reality. The other corners of the figure reflect

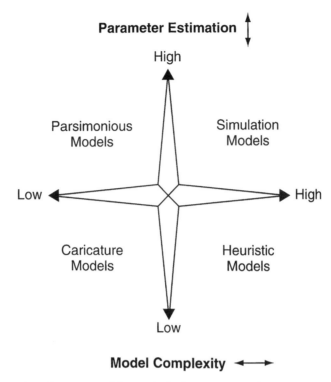

FIGURE 3-9. *The spectrum of mathematic model types for biologic systems. The axes running left to right describe model complexity, and the vertical axes describe the ability of the experimenter to estimate the parameters. Therefore, a highly complex model with many parameters that cannot easily be estimated is heuristic and descriptive, whereas a simple model with few parameters that can be estimated is parsimonious.*

other philosophies in modeling. Parsimonious models are as simple as possible and not expected to describe the experimental situation completely. However, the extent to which the minimal assumptions fail to model reality offers insights into mechanisms. Heuristic models can be extremely complex and, because they usually have a great many parameters, meaningful simulation of data is not possible. However, heuristic models can be useful to define unique behaviors of complex systems which, in turn, can provide insight into the complexity of the biologic system.

The cubic ternary complex model is heuristic and illustrates another feature of receptor systems—namely, that the various species of receptor and receptor-membrane protein complexes that could exist thermodynamically must be considered different with respect to drug binding. Thus, unless α, β, and γ all equal to unity in the preceding model, the binding of a drug to this system will alter the relative distribution of the receptor between the various states of R_i, R_a, $R_i G$, $R_a G$, $AR_i G$, and $AR_a G$. In fact, this becomes a molecular model for drug efficacy, defined as the ability of a drug to alter the interaction of receptors with other proteins in the receptor system. The consequences of these ideas on the observed activity of drugs will be dealt with more fully in Chapter 6.

3.5 THE OPERATIONAL MODEL OF DRUG ACTION

A theoretically more parsimonious model of drug action, termed the *operational model*, was developed by Sir James Black and Paul Leff (11). In this model, the equations stem from the need to describe what is experimentally observed and not necessarily from what is believed to occur on a molecular level. The result provides a mathematic description of experimental datasets from which a resulting molecular mechanism can be deduced.

The initial observation was made that most dose-response curves for drug action are hyperbolic in nature. A mathematic consequence of that observation is that, because the binding of a drug to a receptor is a hyperbolic process, then the relationship between the concentration of drug-receptor complex and response also is hyperbolic. Therefore, the response to a drug (denoted E_a) is given by the following general relationship:

$$E_a = \frac{[A]\,[R_t]\,E_m}{K_A\,K_E + ([R_t] + K_E)[A]} \qquad [3.28]$$

where the concentration of drug is given as $[A]$, the equilibrium dissociation constant of the drug-receptor complex is denoted by K_A, the maximal response is given by E_m, the total concentration of receptors is denoted by $[R_t]$, and the operational fitting parameter that equals the concentration of drug-receptor complex that produces half the maximal response is given as K_E. Black and Leff then defined a transducer constant τ as $[R_t]/K_E$ which described the ability of both the agonist and the system to produce response to the agonist. Thus tissues with high receptor densities or an extremely efficient translation mechanism for the conversion of receptor occupancy into tissue response (i.e., very small K_E such that low concentrations of agonist produce half-maximal responses) had a high transduction capacity for agonism (high τ). Similarly, a highly efficacious drug would impart a large signal to the tissue on receptor occupancy, and this would be reflected in a small value for K_E. Thus, the term K_E characterized *both* the tissue and agonist-specific aspects of efficacy. Under these circumstances, equation 3.28 can be rewritten:

$$\frac{E_a}{E_m} = \frac{[A]\tau}{K_A + (\tau + 1)[A]} \qquad [3.29]$$

This describes agonism as a succession of two hyperbolic functions, the first encompassing the binding of the drug to the receptor and the second the binding of the drug-receptor complex to the stimulus-response machinery of

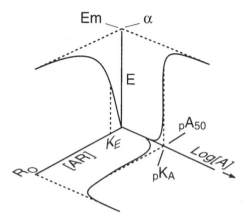

FIGURE 3-10. *The relationship between receptor occupancy and drug concentration (bottom log [A] versus [AR]), between receptor occupancy and response (left face [AR] versus E) and between log dose and response (right face Log [A] versus E), according to the operational model of drug action.*

the tissue to produce observed response (Figure 3-10). It is noteworthy that the operational model does not require an ad hoc constant to describe the efficacy of an agonist. In contrast, the transducer constant τ describes the efficiency with which a given receptor system amplifies receptor stimulus ($[R_t]$ and K_E) and also the intrinsic ability of the agonist to stimulate the receptor (an agonist-specific component of K_E).

The operational model also accounts for a commonly observed phenomenon: when a potent agonist does not produce the tissue maximal response. The maximal asymptote for a drug response can be obtained by setting [A] in Equation 3.29. Under these circumstances, the maximal response to a given agonist is:

$$\underset{(E_a \text{ as}[A]\to\infty)}{\text{Asymptote}} = \frac{E_m\tau}{\tau + 1} \qquad [3.30]$$

Therefore, for agonists of low efficacy (i.e. K_E is large), partial agonism will occur in some tissues (where $[R_t]$ is low) and full agonism in others (where $[R_t]$ is high).

3.6 SYNOPSIS

The following ideas were presented in this chapter:

- Models for the action of drugs have intimated the receptor concept for centuries. Early studies by Langley and Ehrlich defined receptor operationally and, later, Clark defined the theory in mathematic terms.

- Ariens first considered the problem of efficacy. Stephenson introduced the concept of stimulus-response coupling and revolutionized receptor theory.

- Two-state theory also greatly influenced receptor theory; the idea that selective binding of drugs to two interconvertible species could cause shifts in equilibrium steady states of the species offered a molecular basis for efficacy.

- The idea that heterotrimers can be formed from drug-receptor systems also influenced the development of receptor theory. Two-state theory and the idea that receptors can translocate in membranes led to the ternary complex model of membrane drug action.

- The concept of microscopic reversibility and conservation of species can be used to construct mathematic models of any receptor system.

- The operational model of drug action can be used to derive system-independent constants of drug action from functional systems, with no need for the definition of molecular mechanism.

REFERENCES

1. Clark AJ. General pharmacology. In: Heffner's Handbuch d-exp. Pharmacol. Erg. band 4. Berlin:Springer,1937.
2. Parascandola J. The development of receptor theory. In: Parnham MJ, Bruinvels J, eds. Pharmacological methods, receptors and chemotherapy, vol. 3. Amsterdam: Elsevier, 1986: 129–158.
3. Ariens EJ. Molecular pharmacology, Vol 1. New York:Academic Press, 1964.
4. Ariens EJ. Affinity and intrinsic activity in the theory of competitive inhibition. Arch Int Pharmacodyn Ther 1954; 99: 32–49
5. Stephenson RP. A modification of receptor theory. Br J Pharmacol 1956;11:379–393.Black JW, Leff P, Operational models of pharmacological agonists. Proc. Roy. Soc. Lond. (Biol). 1983;220:141–162.
6. Colquhoun D. The relationship between classical and cooperative models for drug action. In: Rang HP, ed. Drug Receptors. Baltimore: University-Park Press,1973:149–182.
7. Cuatrecasas P. Membrane receptors. Annu. Rev. Biochem. 1974;43:169–214.
8. DeLean A, Stadel JM, Lefkowitz RJ. A ternary complex model explains the agonist-specific binding properties of adenylate cyclase coupled β-adrenergic receptor. J Biol Chem 1980;255:7108–7117.
9. Wyman J. The turning wheel: a study in steady states. Proc Natl Acad Sci 1975; 72:3983–3987.
10. Weiss JM, Morgan PH Lutz MW Kenakin TP. The cubic ternary complex receptor

occupancy model: II. Understanding apparent affinity. J Theoret Biol 1996; 178: 151–182.

11. Black JW, Leff P. Operational models of pharmacological agonists. Proc R Soc Lond Biol Sci 1983;220:141–162.

FURTHER READING

Onaran HO, Costa T, Rodbard D. βγ subunits of guanine nucleotide-binding proteins and regulation of spontaneous receptor activity: Thermodynamic model for the interaction between receptors and guanine nucleotide-binding protein subunits. Mol. Pharmacol 1993;43:245–256.

Samama P, Cotecchia S, Costa T, Lefkowitz RJ. A mutation-induced activated state of the β_2-adrenergic receptor: Extending the ternary complex model. J. Biol. Chem. 1993;268:4625–4636.

Human Receptors from Recombinant DNA

I N THIS CHAPTER is described the use of molecular biology for the creation of human receptor systems. In previous years, the lack of access to human receptors has necessitated the use of animal receptor systems in pharmacology and drug discovery. With the advent of techniques allowing the introduction of human genetic material encoding for receptors into surrogate cell lines has come a new age in pharmacology. Section 4.1 lists the advantages of this approach. Section 4.2 discusses human genes and the construction of genetic libraries. Genetic material is introduced, via carriers (vectors), into bacterial cells, where the material is separated into pure colonies (clones) and replicates. The resulting genetic product then is transfected into surrogate cells to form cell clones containing human receptors suitable for pharmacologic research. Section 4.3 through 4.6 introduce molecular biologic techniques useful in the study of receptors and the creation of genetically engineered receptor systems . The synopsis touches on the major ideas discussed in the chapter (section 4.7).

4.1 WHY USE RECOMBINANT SYSTEMS?

Progress in the field of molecular biology has furnished the ability physically to construct receptor systems for the testing of drugs as well as for the detailed study of human receptors. Previously, pharmacology was constrained to the study of animal receptor systems, the rationale for correspondence to human systems being that many of the molecules mediating responses via these receptors (e.g., neurotransmitters such as acetylcholine, hormones such as epinephrine) were the same in animals and in humans. Therefore, a correspondence was anticipated between the recognition sites for these molecules (receptors) in the two species. Though most of the known therapeutic drugs in use today were discovered using such systems, it is clear that they are facsimiles of the therapeutic target system. Table 4-1 shows the various drug receptor systems that can be used for drug discovery. The development of new drugs is considerably advanced by the ability to use human target receptors in controlled testing systems.

With the advent of the cloning of the first bacteriorhodopsin in the 1980s has come the ability to introduce the genetic material that codes for human receptors into appropriate surrogate host cells for study in isolation. Furthermore, these surrogate host systems can be human cells, to provide a more physiologic environment. However, in numerous cases the specific cell type in which the human receptor resides in nature exerts an important influence on the behavior of receptors and this is lost in a surrogate system. Furthermore, pathologic processes can have important and, in some cases, dominant influences on human receptor function. Therefore, though genetic engineering can do much to improve the design of receptor systems, it still often falls short of the objective namely, that of producing a human receptor in its native human cell under pathologic control.

There are basically three reasons for constructing receptor systems with molecular biology. The first is the obvious access to human, rather than animal, receptor material. The second is that many physiologic systems design

---

TABLE 4-1 Chronology of Drug Receptor Systems Used in Drug Discovery

---

Animal receptors, animal tissues

Animal or human cells in culture

Animal genetic receptor material, surrogate cells

Human genetic receptor material, surrogate cells

Human receptors, human target cell

Human receptors, human target cell (appropriate pathologic control)

---

backup control of receptor systems for fine-tuning of response to chemicals. Thus, many cells express mixtures of receptor subtypes that differ subtly one from another with respect to recognition and translation of pharmacologic and physiologic information. This poses a practical problem for those who wish to study drug-receptor interaction, because the responses are mediated by multiple, rather than single, receptor populations. The genetic engineering of a receptor system can eliminate this by expressing a single receptor population in a surrogate cell that otherwise does not contain the receptor, thus allowing the study of drug effect on a single receptor population.

The third reason for genetically constructing a receptor system is to gain the ability to answer questions about the receptor itself. One obvious area is the overproduction of receptor material for isolation and characterization by biochemical means (receptors are found in minute amounts in nature). Another is control of the stoichiometric ratio between receptors and their membrane-bound interactants. With molecular biology, the components of these heterotrimeric systems can be manipulated, thereby furnishing information never before accessible. This can help determine to what extent the activity of a drug is due to its interaction with the system components and to what extent it is unique to the molecular nature of the receptor and the drug. This is important because only the latter features (expressed as receptor-related affinity and efficacy) are transferable between systems. Because the systems used for screening drugs necessarily are different from those to be encountered in therapy, fewer surprises will result with increased knowledge of system-independent drug characteristics.

4.2 CLONING GENES FOR HUMAN RECEPTORS

Genetic information is stored in coded form in structured helices of *deoxyribonucleic acid (DNA)*. Specific sequences of the nucleotides that make up the DNA molecule are read by nuclear mechanisms in the cell, and the transcription and translation of this coded information results in protein synthesis. For the purposes of the molecular pharmacology of drugs and receptors, the focus of this discussion will be the use of *genes* (the section of the chromosome that contains sufficient information to make a specific protein) that code for human receptors. These genes can be *cloned* (production of identical genes from a single individual by asexual processes) and transfected into a host cell to produce a viable human receptor system suitable for the testing of drugs.

The first step is the cloning of the receptor gene. In general, a library of genetic material is made from the target cell, and the components of this library are manipulated into a form suitable for handling. Specifically, the genetic material is placed into a vector of DNA with special properties. The receptor gene DNA and the vector DNA form *recombinant DNA,* which is

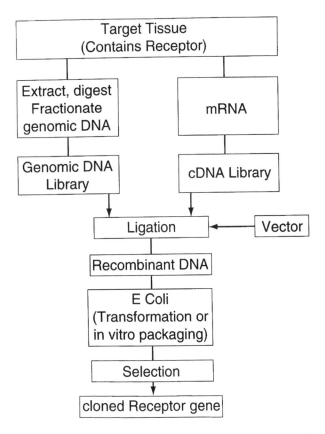

FIGURE 4-1. *Schematic diagram depicting the process of gene cloning. Either genomic DNA or mRNA (which is converted to cDNA) is isolated from the tissue and ligated into a vector. The resulting recombinant DNA is placed into bacterial cells, and the thus transformed bacteria is selected from untransformed cells.*

suitable for cloning cells (usually bacteria such as *Escherichia coli*). The recombinant DNA is multiplied as the cells form *clones* (colonies). Each cell in the colony carries an identical copy of the recombinant DNA; thus the gene is said to be *cloned*. The colonies are screened for selection of the recombinant DNA of interest, and these are used subsequently to produce the cellular receptor system. The general procedure is shown schematically in Figure 4-1.

4.2.1 Libraries

The complete DNA of an organism can be quantified in terms of nucleic acid base pairs, the rungs on the DNA ladder coding for proteins. The number of base pairs for organisms varies widely from 4 million for *E. coli*, 700 million for a tomato, and 3 billion for a human. In terms of cloning a human receptor, a receptor gene therefore may comprise one part in 2 million. The key to obtaining a particular gene is to ensure a huge population of DNA portions that represent every gene of the organism (or at least every gene transcribed in the target tissue). The first step in this process is the construction of a *library* (fragments of DNA) of genetic material from an appropriate cell. For example, if a particular receptor for human diabetes is the target, then an appropriate cell from which to make a library might be a human β pancreatic cell (secretion of insulin). *Genomic DNA* consists of the complete DNA from a cell severed in random pieces with restriction endonucleases. Though the complete genetic code of the organism is contained in this library (the *genome*), the gene of interest may be difficult to isolate.

There are several practical reasons for making another type of library—a *complementary DNA (cDNA)* library—from the host cell genetic material. Discussion of these types of libraries requires discussion of the process of DNA transcription. Protein synthesis occurs when the genetic code of a portion of the DNA helix is used by the enzyme RNA polymerase to make a corresponding coded molecule called *ribonucleic acid (RNA)*. Because the code comes from a particular gene coding for a specific protein and the RNA transcribes this code and carries it to a large and complex subcellular molecular machine known as a *ribosome* for translation into a protein sequence, the RNA is referred to as *messenger RNA (mRNA)*. Of note is the fact that for every protein synthesized in the cell (including receptors), there is a correspondingly unique mRNA. In highly differentiated cells, the mRNA for a particular protein may represent up to 10% or more of the total RNA, while rare messages may exist in a ratio of only 1 in 1 million.

Only a fraction of the total genome is transcribed into RNA. However, there are advantages to cloning a cDNA library for the isolation of particular receptors. First, mRNA exists for proteins actively synthesized by the cell. Therefore, if the receptor of interest is known to exist naturally in the cell from which the library is to be made, then the mRNA for that protein may exist in high quantities (greater than the single gene in the genome). Also, there are practical considerations, such as ease of purification and isolation of mRNA, that favor cDNA library production.

A copy of the piece of DNA from which the mRNA was transcribed can be made from the mRNA. First, a single strand of DNA is made from the mRNA by the enzyme reverse transcriptase. The resulting single-stranded DNA forms a hairpin structure, thereby providing a primer for the synthesis of a complementary strand of DNA to be made by DNA polymerase. Another method of making cDNA from mRNA is with the enzyme R Nase H, from *E. coli,* which recognizes RNA-DNA hybrids and digests the RNA into short pieces. These pieces remain hybridized to the first DNA strand and serve as hybrids for *E. coli* DNA polymerase I, which synthesizes double-stranded DNA from the original DNA template. The result of either of these processes is a piece of double-stranded cDNA containing the genetic material to produce the protein of interest.

4.2.2 DNA Vectors

Once the cDNA is produced it must be introduced into a carrier, or vector, that will cause entry into the host cell nuclear machinery. The discovery of restriction endonucleases and ligases, two enzymes that cut and paste DNA segments respectively, has allowed DNA fragments to be manipulated and fused with other DNA to produce small double-stranded circular portions of DNA called *plasmids*. Thus, the DNA fragment of interest (to be termed the *passenger DNA*) is linked to a carrier vector DNA (which itself possesses a number of genes) to form a unit (recombinant DNA) with special properties for the cloning of the passenger DNA. Useful vectors contain a region of DNA capable of functioning as an origin of replication that will allow it to multiply independently in the host. Vectors also contain promoters, which are DNA sequences that direct the synthesis of large amounts of mRNA corresponding to the gene. In addition, they can include sequences to increase the efficiency with which the mRNA is translated. Finally, they contain one or more genes to confer antibiotic resistance to the host. This latter property functions as a marker for the cells containing the plasmid to be isolated (i.e., the cell culture is treated with the antibiotic and only the successfully transfected cells will live because they possess antibiotic resistance). Ideally, they should contain a second selectable gene that is inactivated by insertion of the passenger DNA, as this greatly assists in the selection process. This allows for the separation of cells transformed by plasmids that do not have successfully incorporated passenger DNA (Fig 4-2A).

4.2.3 Bacterial Cell Transformation and Selection

The next step in the cloning procedure is to introduce the plasmids containing the passenger DNA into a cell that will allow it to replicate. Bacterial cells, and in particular *E. coli*, are ideally suited for this as they are easy to manipulate and can grow rapidly in inexpensive media. Most bacteria take up only limited quantities of DNA; therefore, they must be treated physically or chemically to give them enhanced properties for uptake of DNA (i.e., the cells must be transformed). Cells are made competent to take up DNA by soaking in cold, 50-mM calcium chloride (or rubidium chloride) solution. This causes the DNA to adhere to the outer cell wall. A brief heat shock (e.g., 42°C for 2 minutes) causes the DNA to be transported into the cytoplasm.

Cells are transfected with a collection of plasmids from the cDNA library at such a concentration to allow only one plasmid to enter a single cell. In effect, the passenger DNA is now in its own little factory where, as that particular cell divides into a colony, numerous copies of the passenger will divide with it and a clone of the recombinant DNA will be made with the colony. Thus, a few nanograms of recombinant DNA can become several micrograms (thousands-

Clone Selection

A. BR322 Plasmid

B. Replica Plating

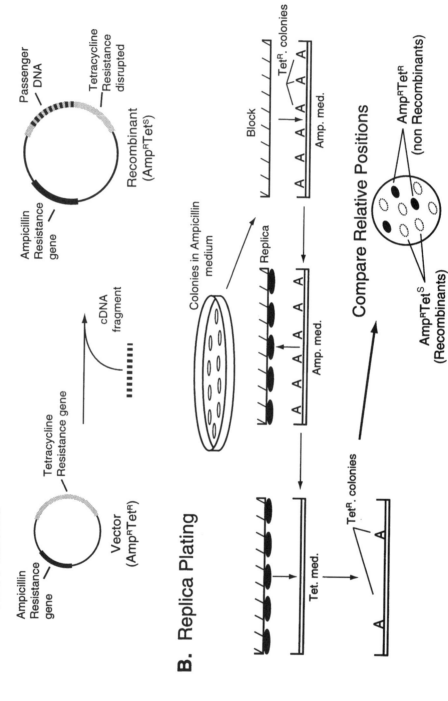

fold increase) in a single bacterial culture. However, although 1000 to 10,000 transformants can be made in a culture, this represents only a small fraction of the total cell population. The next step is amplification of the transformed cells over non-transformed cells, which is accomplished with the selection genes built into the cloning vector. Thus, cells containing a vector that possesses a gene to impart a resistance to antibacterial drug (e.g., the plasmid RP4 contains genes to impart resistance to ampicillin, kanamycin, and tetracycline) will be immune to these drugs. Therefore, treatment of the complete culture with tetracycline will kill cells not containing plasmid, leaving the *recombinants* (those successfully transformed with plasmid) to thrive.

Another feature of vectors, known as *insertional inactivation,* can select further for successful recombinants. This is useful for selecting out those cells that take up plasmid only with no corresponding passenger DNA (i.e., remove plasmid transformed *versus* recombinant DNA transformed). To accomplish this, the vector can have more than one gene for antibiotic resistance, with one of the genes having unique restriction sites suitable to open and insert passenger DNA. If this is done, then the plasmid recombinant with passenger DNA will lose the particular resistance corresponding to the disrupted gene, which allows for the selection not only of cells that are transformed by plasmid but also of those cells that carry successfully inserted passenger DNA in the plasmid by a process known as *replicate plating* (see Fig 4-2B).

4.2.4 Transfection of Cells

In terms of producing a recombinant human receptor system suitable for the testing of drugs and for investigation of receptor mechanisms, the receptor gene must be cloned into a surrogate cellular host. The first step in this process is the *transfection* of the recombinant DNA into the host cell. Most mammalian transfection vectors use cDNA fragments as opposed to genomic DNA. Useful vectors contain multiple elements to an origin of amplification,

---

FIGURE 4-2. *The selection of clones. A. Example of a plasmid (BR322 plasmid) used for gene cloning. Two genes conferring bacterial resistance (ampicillin and tetracycline) are present in the plasmid. When a passenger cDNA is introduced into the plasmid, the gene for tetracycline resistance (Tet^R) is disrupted. Thus, cells with a plasmid containing the cDNA are ampicillin- resistant (Amp^R) but tetracycline-sensitive (Tet^S). B. Replica plating as a means of clone selection. Cells containing clones are grown in ampicillin medium, thereby selecting for plasmid-containing bacteria (ampicillin-resistant). A wooden block is pressed into the culture to form a replica of the cell colonies; these are replicated in a tetracycline-containing medium, which leaves the colonies resistant to tetracycline only (i.e., the clones contain the plasmid without the cDNA as the tetracycline gene has not been disrupted). The imprinted block then is compared to the original culture plate, thus identifying the colonies transfected with non-cDNA-containing plasmid. The ampicillin-resistant but tetracycline-sensitive cells contain the gene of interest.*

an efficient promoter for high-level transcription, and suitable markers for selection. Vectors also can contain an inducible expression system that can be controlled by external stimuli. Under these circumstances, stimuli such as β-interferon, heatshock, heavy-metal ions, and steroids can be used to control the level of expression of the protein coded by the passenger gene. A number of methods exist for introducing transfection vectors into mammalian cells such as treatment of cells with calcium phosphate, DEAE-dextran transfection, electroporation (high voltage electric field that form temporary holes in membrane), and liposome-mediated transfection.

In addition to plasmid transfection of recombinant DNA into cells, viral transfer also can be accomplished. Viruses such as the SV40 recombinant virus, retroviruses, and vaccinia virus can infect many cell types and thus allow the opportunity to inject foreign genes efficiently. Some of these systems (baculovirus, vaccinia virus) produce overexpression of protein and so can be used to attain high expression levels. The baculovirus, in particular, is useful as it utilizes insect cells that process protein in much the same way as higher eukaryotic cells (myristylation, palmitoylation, glycosylation, etc.). Included in the genome for this virus, which does not infect vertebrates, is a gene for a protein that exists in the host in large crystalline bodies, making up 50% of the cell. Replacement of this gene with a foreign one allows similar production of the protein of interest with relative ease.

In general, the process of gene cloning is complete when a single gene has been identified, isolated, and amplified. The cloning of a particular gene can be thought of as the isolation of a particular piece of DNA (uptake of the passenger DNA ligated into a cloning vector into a single cell), the replication of that particular gene within the isolated environment, and the identification of the particular clone of interest by selection (Summary shown in Fig 4-3).

4.2.5 Transient and Stable Clones

Two types of transfection, *transient* and *stable*, normally are performed in mammalian systems. Transient transfection allows analysis of protein product within 1 to 4 days of transfection. The efficiency of transient transfection depends on the number of cells that take up the foreign DNA, the gene copy number, and the expression level per gene. In general, as much as 50% and as little as 5% of the cells take up recombinant DNA transiently. Because the cells that do take up the foreign DNA grow more slowly than other cells, eventually they are lost from the population. Therefore, the transiently transfected cells carry the recombinant DNA signal for periods of several days to a maximum of a few weeks. Transient transfection is difficult to scale up for production of large amounts of protein, but it is a convenient method for testing functionality of plasmid and, especially relevant to the study of human drug receptors, it is used for expression cloning (*vide infra*).

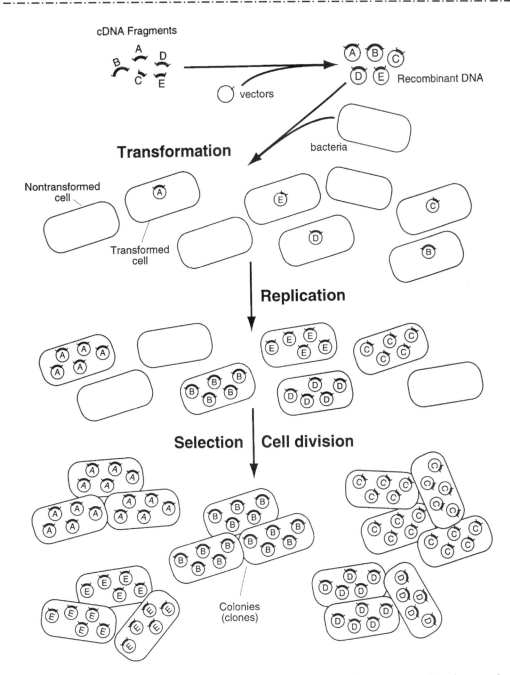

FIGURE 4-3. *The cloning of a gene. DNA fragments A to E are inserted into vectors and used to transform bacterial cells. One cell takes up a single plasmid. The cells containing plasmid make numerous copies of the plasmid and replicate into colonies. The process of selection isolates a colony of cells containing numerous copies of the DNA of interest. This gene is thus isolated and replicated.*

Approximately 1 in 10^4 cells (in some systems, as much as 1 in 1000) in a transfection will stably integrate the foreign DNA into their chromosomal DNA and thus express the protein as native throughout its life cycle. Unlike transient expression in which efficiency depends on DNA uptake, the efficiency of stable transfection depends on the frequency of DNA integration. If selection for these stably transfected cells is made, then a colony expressing the gene of interest can be obtained after approximately 10 doublings; from this, an individual colony can be chosen and grown into a stable cell line. This cell line then will consistently express the product of the cloned gene as part of its natural makeup. Selection uses the principle of conference of drug resistance to hosts deficient in the particular activity selected. Therefore, if a marker gene is cotransfected into the cell with the recombinant gene of interest in a ratio of 1:5 (one part marker and five parts recombinant gene of interest), this effectively ensures that every cell containing marker gene also will contain the gene of interest. This can also be accomplished by building the marker gene into the plasmid containing the gene of interest.

Selection markers can be highly varied. For example, a marker gene could code for the enzyme adenosine deaminase (ADA), which detoxifies Xyl-A (9-b-D-xylofuranosyl adenine) to its inosine derivative. If Xyl-A is not detoxified, it is converted to Xyl-ATP, which is toxic to the cell. Therefore, ADA-deficient CHO cells can be used to select for transfection. Similarly, a gene for aminoglycoside phosphotransferase (APH) can produce a cell resistant to the protein synthesis blocker G418. Under these circumstances, transfected cells grown in G418 will survive, whereas untransfected cells will die.

Cells are transfected and cultured through the transient phase. With further culture, transiently transfected cells die leaving the much lower complement of cells (1 in 10^4) that have incorporated the foreign DNA into their chromosome (stably transfected). Then, the selection media (Xyl-A for ADA marker, G418 for APH marker, etc.) is added, which kills untransfected cells, leaving the stably transfected cells to proliferate (Fig 4-4).

Stable cell lines containing human receptors are the ultimate goal of the molecular biology described in this chapter. However, a number of issues related to receptor pharmacology can be addressed by molecular biology.

4.3 EXPRESSION CLONING OF RECEPTORS

The preceding discussion involved the cloning of a gene and creation of a cellular system carrying pure amounts of the product of that gene. However, if the code for the particular receptor is not known, the only marker available to detect cloning of the appropriate gene is the receptor activity itself. Under these conditions, cDNA libraries are transfected into cells that then are subjected to pharmacologic analysis for receptor function; this is referred to as

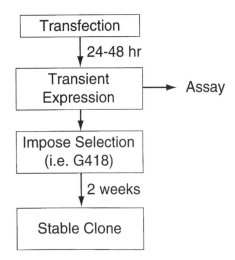

FIGURE 4-4. *The production of stable clones. Cells are transfected with plasmid and, within 24 to 48 hours, a certain proportion have expressed the gene product. A very small proportion of the cells have incorporated the foreign DNA into their own DNA, and these subsequently are amplified. Selection is imposed (i.e., G418 or Xyl-A medium) and, in approximately 2 weeks, a stable colony of the cells containing the foreign gene results.*

expression cloning. For example, the receptor for a hypothetical neural brain hormone may be known to be highly localized in a certain area of the brain (e.g., the hypothalamus). In this instance, it would be reasonable to assume that the hypothalamic cells would possess a certain quantity of mRNA for that receptor, as the receptor is known to be localized in those cells. Therefore, a cDNA library could be made and used to transfect host cells. The library could then be divided into pools of cDNA and used to transfect multiple culture plates of mammalian cellular hosts. These, in turn, could be screened for receptor by radioligand binding or receptor function. For the purposes of this discussion, the process is simply one of selection of a positive pool. The determination of a positive receptor signal in one of the plates means that only one of thousands or so genes in that aliquot is the correct one. The process is repeated to narrow the choices down to a single gene. The plasmid cDNA is pooled from the positive culture plate and is used to culture another set of plates. The positive plate again is isolated, and the process is repeated such that a single plate is divided into colony regions and then into single colonies until a clone is obtained (Fig 4-5). The plasmid cDNA from this single clone contains the gene for the specific receptor of interest. From here, it can be introduced into a number of cellular hosts for exploratory research and into baculovirus for high production of receptor protein. Furthermore, the DNA can be sequenced and the receptor amino acid sequence of the receptor determined.

Expression Cloning of Receptors

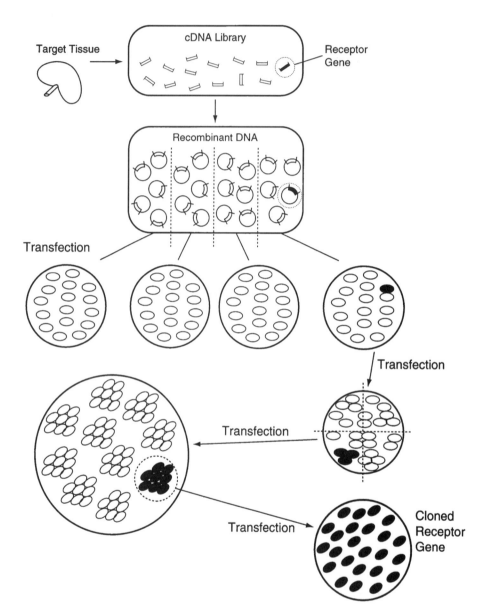

FIGURE 4-5. *The process of expression cloning. A library is constructed from a target tissue, made into recombinant DNA, and divided into pools. The separate pools are used to transfect separate cell cultures, and each is assayed for gene product (i.e., receptor presence by radioligand binding, functional response to agonist). DNA from the active culture is used to transfect a fresh culture, which then is divided into sections and reassayed. The process continues until the specific cell colony containing cells expressing the gene product is isolated.*

4.4 DNA TO PROTEIN SEQUENCE: THE GENETIC CODE

As mentioned earlier in this chapter, DNA contains coded sequences of nucleic acids that provide the recipe for construction of designated amino acids into proteins. DNA is made up of four nucleic acids, thymine, adenine, cytosine, and guanine that form stable hybrid pairs with one another (thymine to adenine and cytosine to guanine; Fig 4-6A). The precise order of the amino acids determines the nature and structure of the protein, and this precise order is contained in the arrangement of nucleic acids in the helices of the DNA molecule (see Fig 4-6B). The bases must code for 20 different amino acids. It can be seen from this arrangement that a single nucleic acid could not code for 1 protein (only 4 could be coded), nucleic acid pairs could only code for 16 amino acids, and 3 amino acids could code for 64 amino acids. The actual code is a triplet (shown in Fig 4-7), and it can be seen that a number of triplets code for more than one amino acid, whereas some triplets are stop codons (signal the end of synthesis). The relevance to receptor research is the fact that knowledge of the nucleic acid sequence of receptor cDNA can be used to back-translate the amino acid sequence of the receptor. Therefore, knowledge of the gene sequence of a receptor leads to knowledge about the protein sequence.

Another important aspect of the correspondence between nucleic and amino acids is the construction of oligonucleotide probes to isolate clones and search for subtypes and mutants of receptors. A powerful method to isolate and identify a particular clone of interest is by nucleic acid hybridization (*colony hybridization*). The colonies of cells, spread on agarose plates, are imprinted with a nitrocellulose or nylon membrane such that a replica of the plate is made with a few of the cells. The membrane is treated to remove all material but DNA, which then is fixed to the membrane in the exact position of the colony from whence it came by heating. A probe then is used to identify the colony containing the recombinant of interest. Some probes are radioactive and can be detected by autoradiography, but another type of probe uses biotin, which can be detected with a tight binding to the protein avidin (detected with fluorescent dyes such as Texas red).

The principle on which this is based is that nucleic acids of complementary structure will bind to one another and form hybrid structures as they do in the DNA helix (*vide infra*). Therefore, if a portion of the nucleic acid sequence of the gene of interest is known, then the collection of bacterial cell colonies could be exposed to a selectable (i.e., either radioactive or biotin-containing) complementary probe and allow identification of the colony containing that gene. The key element in this process is having the correct probe, as colony hybridization requires a unique sequence of radioactive nucleotides that will hybridize to a unique portion of the cDNA and allow isolation. For example, Figure 4-8A shows a sequence of DNA from a receptor

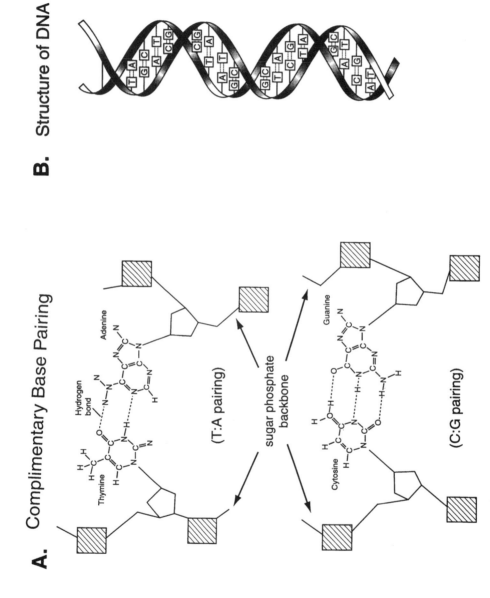

A. Complimentary Base Pairing

B. Structure of DNA

FIGURE 4-6. *The DNA molecule. A. Specific pairing of complementary bases in the DNA strand. Thymine binds to adenine, and cytosine binds to guanine. B. The individual base pairing across the two strands of DNA leads to the alpha helix structure.*

THE GENETIC CODE

FIRST POSITION	SECOND POSITION				THIRD POSITION
	T	C	A	G	
T	PHE	SER	TYR	CYS	T
	PHE	SER	TYR	CYS	C
	LEU	SER	stop	stop	A
	LEU	SER	stop	TRP	G
T	LEU	PRO	HIS	ARG	T
	LEU	PRO	HIS	ARG	C
	LEU	PRO	GLN	ARG	A
	LEU	PRO	GLN	ARG	G
A	ILE	THR	ASN	SER	T
	ILE	THR	LYS	SER	C
	ILE	THR	LYS	ARG	A
	MET	THR	LYS	ARG	G
G	VAL	ALA	ASP	GLY	T
	VAL	ALA	ASP	GLY	C
	VAL	ALA	GLU	GLY	A
	VAL	ALA	GLU	GLY	G

NUCLEIC ACIDS
A= adenine   **C**= cytosine   **G**= guanine   **T**= Thymine

Amino ACIDS
GLY= glycine   **ALA**= alanine   **VAL**= valine   **LEU**= leucine
ILE= isoleucine   **SER**= serine   **CYS**= cysteine   **MET**= methionine
TYR= tyrosine   **PHE**= phenylalanine   **TRP**= tryptophan   **HIS**= histidine
ARG= arginine   **LYS**= lysine   **ASP**= aspartic acid   **GLU**= glutamic acid
ASN= asparagine   **GLN**= glutamine   **PRO**= proline   **THR**= threonine

FIGURE 4-7. *The genetic code. Triplet bases along the DNA strand code for a given amino acid. Degeneracy occurs (i.e., four triplets all code for proline), and stop codons signal when translation should end.*

gene and the corresponding amino acid sequence for which it codes. Consider the reverse problem, the design of a nucleic acid probe for this particular amino acid sequence. Because of degeneracy in the genetic code (i.e., many amino acids are coded for by more than one triplet sequence), the possible nucleic acid sequences that could correspond to the protein sequence are shown (see Fig 4-8B); in this particular case, four. Hybrids are formed be-

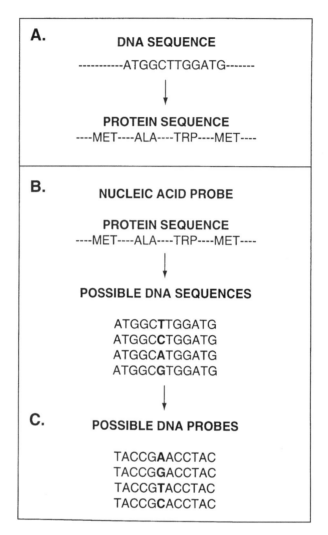

FIGURE 4-8. *Oligonucleotide probes. A. Sequence of 12 base codes for four amino acids in the gene of interest. B. This protein sequence can be coded for four different oligonucleotide sequences according to the genetic code (note degeneracy for ALA). C. The complementary probes that can bind to the sequence of interest are synthesized and can be used to detect the original gene.*

tween the nucleic acids adenine and thymine and also between guanine and cytosine. The four probes that would hybridize to the four sequences are shown in Figure 4-8C. For colony hybridization, a mixture of these four oligonucleotides would be made and used to screen for the particular receptor gene. Clearly, the degeneracy in the genetic code can lead to considerable ambiguity if amino acid sequences are chosen for which there are many possible nucleic acid codes. For example, the sequence —VAL—LEU— ARG—LEU— has 864 possible oligonucleotide sequences, clearly a less than useful portion of the protein for a unique probe. In general, a sequence containing amino acids that are coded for histidine or asparagine is useful because only a single triplet codes for these amino acids.

Probes can be less stringent for sequences by design. For example, different receptors share areas of homology (similar amino acid sequences), thereby offering the opportunity of using an oligonucleotide for one type of receptor to probe for the gene to another kind of receptor. Similarly, a limited amino acid sequence can select a gene for a *receptor subtype,* one produced by the host cell, which has slight amino acid differences from the normal receptor (Fig 4-9). Such receptors can be produced by pathologic processes (i.e.,

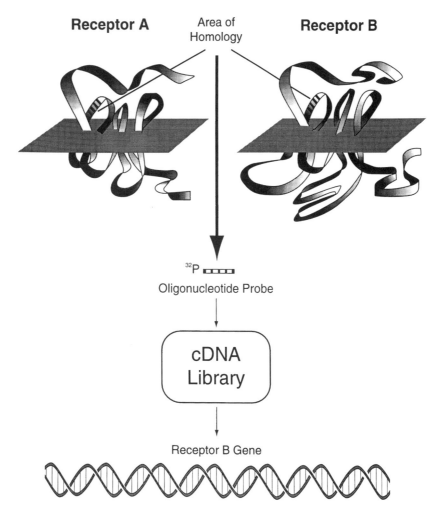

FIGURE 4-9. *Use of sequence homology to detect similar receptors. Two receptors are different except for certain stretches of amino acids that are the same (homologous regions). An oligonucleotide probe coding for this region can be used to isolate the original receptor (A) and other receptors containing this same sequence (receptor B).*

cancer or other diseases). Discoveries of this sort can be extremely important as they present the opportunity to design selective drugs for new receptors.

4.5 THE POLYMERASE CHAIN REACTION (PCR)

Another technique in molecular biology, the polymerase chain reaction (PCR), is extremely useful for the detection of genes in libraries and, therefore, for the mapping of genes for receptors in different tissues. As noted previously, DNA exists as a double helix of hybridized base pairs (adenine to thymine and guanine to cytosine). However, these strands can be denatured chemically or by heat into single strands. From these single strands, new copies of corresponding DNA can be made by the enzyme DNA polymerase. The complementary strand to each separate strand is made, so that when these are renatured again, a copy of the original DNA strand results. Repetition of the reaction can produce prodigious copies of a single piece of DNA. This technique makes use of the fact that the enzyme DNA polymerase requires a primer (small string of nucleotides) to which it can add bases to form strands of DNA. This primer hybridizes to a specific part of the DNA to be amplified, and new DNA synthesis begins from this point. Therefore, if the precise starting point of a gene sequence is known, then a primer can be synthesized to bind to that precise point to begin synthesis. Thus, by denaturation of the DNA sample and addition of an excess amount of two primers that represent sequences framing the gene of interest, multiple copies of the gene can be manufactured (shown schematically in Fig 4-10). The number of copies of the gene equals $(2^n)/4$, where n is the number of times the PCR is run. For example, a gene can be made into 1 million copies by performing the reaction 22 times. This offers tremendous power of detection of genes because PCR can be run with appropriate primers for different receptors and the presence of that same gene in any tissue can be detected.

PCR is a very powerful technique, capable of detecting a single piece of DNA in a complete library. One application of this technology is the detection of receptor mutants. The genetic information about such mutants often is sparse as the mutation may limit the production of the host. However, mutant receptors can be important in the structural and functional changes that accompany some diseases, and the testing of new drug entities on mutant receptors is desirable. With PCR, the limiting coding regions for receptors can be defined, and all DNA corresponding to the coding between those start codons will be amplified. If a receptor point mutation is present, this too will be amplified, such that large quantities can be made and sequenced (Fig 4-11). Expression cloning of the mutant receptor then would be possible with subsequent pharmacologic testing.

Polymerase Chain Reaction

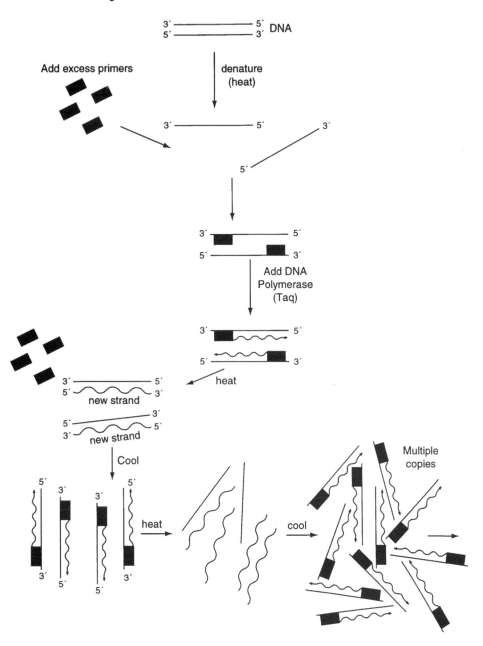

FIGURE 4-10. *The polymerase chain reaction. The DNA is denatured to separate the chains, and an excess of primers that will bind to the two regions on the DNA that define the gene of interest is added. The primers bind to the boundary areas of the gene and function as a template for DNA polymerase to begin synthesis of complementary strands. The chains are separated by heat and the process repeated; thus, every new synthesized DNA strand functions as a template for further copies. With each repeat process, new DNA accumulates.*

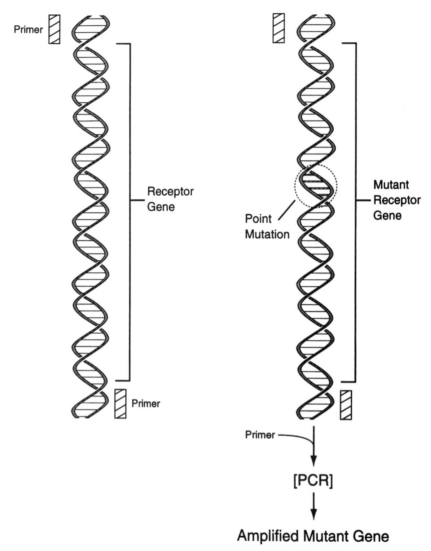

FIGURE 4-11. *The use of the polymerase chain reaction (PCR) to detect receptor mutation. The primers define a gene that may have a point mutation. This mutated gene would still be amplified by the PCR technique.*

4.6 GENETICALLY ENGINEERED RECEPTOR SYSTEMS

The ability to express gene products in different types of cells has created a revolution in receptor research. This is because receptors do not function in isolation but rather are part of complex interdependent systems (i.e., review the cubic ternary complex model, Chapter 3). Under these circumstances, the molecular nature of the components and their relative stoichiometries affect their behavior and the behavior of drugs on them. In nature, the stoichiometries of receptor systems are tightly controlled according to the needs of the cell and the strength of the chemical input to those cells. Therefore, little latitude has allowed researchers who must depend on judicious choice of natural systems for optimum conditions for drug testing. With the advent of molecular biology, test systems can be created to meet the needs of researchers. The genetic manipulation of cellular components offers a new method of probing these test systems.

4.6.1 Applications of Genetically Controlled Receptor Systems

There are three distinct applications of genetic control of receptor systems as it pertains to receptor research. The *first* is *to control system responsiveness* to detect drug efficacy. It is well-known that a drug with low efficacy may produce no response in an inefficiently coupled receptor system. This can be dissimulating if the drug is intended for use as an antagonist and produces agonist responses in well-coupled tissues in the human body. One method of controlling responsiveness of a receptor system is to control the stoichiometry of the reactants. Thus, different promoters can be used to express various levels of receptor protein or G-protein. Also, coexpression of both receptor and G-protein can be used to create responsive receptor systems. The reaction between receptor (R), G-protein (G), and drug (A) can simplistically be viewed as:

$$[A] + [R] \underset{k_{\text{back}}}{\overset{k_{\text{forward}}}{\rightleftharpoons}} [A \cdot R] + [G] \underset{k'_{\text{back}}}{\overset{k'_{\text{forward}}}{\rightleftharpoons}} [A \cdot R \cdot G] \qquad [4.1]$$

where k_{forward} and k_{back} refer to the rate constants for the forward and backward chemical reactions, respectively. Agonist response is mediated by the formation of the ternary complex $A \cdot R \cdot G$ which in turn is governed by the production of $A \cdot R$. The rate of formation of $A \cdot R$ is given by $k_{\text{forward}}[A][R]$ and that of $A \cdot R \cdot G$ by $k_{\text{forward}}[G][A \cdot R]$. It can be seen from these kinetic reactions that increases in the amount of reactants $[R]$ and $[G]$ will increase the production of the response producing element $A \cdot R \cdot G$. Figure 4.12 shows the effects of increasing either receptor expression level or G-protein level in expression systems on the response-forming ($A \cdot R \cdot G$) ability of an agonist. Two phases, in terms of the changes produced by such manipulation, can be observed. The first is an increase in the maximal asymptote of the dose-response curve (phase I). It should be noted that, depending on the nature and number of intervening steps between the observed response and production of $A \cdot R \cdot G$, there may or may not be a change in the location parameter (median effective concentration [EC_{50}]) of the curves in phase I. In the second phase, the maximal asymptote reaches a plateau and the dose-response curves shift to the left, with increasing expression of either receptor or G-protein. This is because one or more of the components of the system are saturated. For

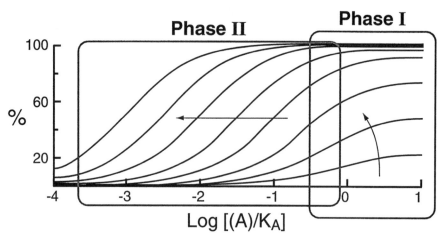

FIGURE 4-12. *The effects of increasing response capability in a functional system. The first observation is an increase in the maximal asymptote response, which may or may not be accompanied by a shift to the left of the EC_{50} of the dose-response curve (phase I). After saturation of one or more of the components of the system, sinistral shifts of the dose-response curves with no change in the maximal response are observed (phase II).*

example, if G-protein levels are increased beyond the stoichiometric equivalent of receptor, then no further maximal $A \cdot R \cdot G$ can be formed (the amount of R limits this), but the probability of forming the complex increases because of increased availability of the reactants. Thus, phase II consists of parallel shifts to the left of the dose-response curve. An example of the changes in sensitivity to an agonist with increasing concentrations of G-protein in a system with a fixed amount of receptor was given in Chapter 3 (see Fig 3-5).

Another reason for manipulating the stoichiometry of a receptor system is to make it constitutively active. Receptors are reactive proteins with many tertiary conformations. Some of these conformations activate G-proteins, thus, they telegraph their presence. In most natural systems, the quantity of spontaneously activated receptor is extremely low, as signaling subject to external stimuli is better controlled under normal physiologic circumstances. However, if the stoichiometry of the receptor and G-proteins is elevated sufficiently, beyond natural limits or in specialized host cells, then an observable level of the spontaneously activated receptor will be produced. This will, in turn, produce a measurable signal in the cell due to an abnormally high level of spontaneously active receptor. Thus, a simplified system for the coexistence of an inactive (R_i) and active (R_a) receptor in the presence of G-protein (G) is expressed as follows:

$$
\begin{array}{ccccc}
[R_i] & + & [G] & \overset{K'_G}{\rightleftharpoons} & [R_iG] \\
\| L & & & & \| \beta L \\
[R_a] & + & [G] & \underset{\beta K'_G}{\rightleftharpoons} & [R_aG]
\end{array}
\qquad [4.2]
$$

where L is the allosteric association constant defined by $[R_a]/[R_i]$, K'_G is the association constant for the receptor and G-protein, and β is a multiplicative factor denoting the difference in the affinity of the active versus the inactive form of the receptor for the G-protein. It is assumed that no cellular response emanates from a nonproductive complex of inactive receptor and G-protein (R_iG), only from the active receptor G-protein complex (R_aG).

The level of R_aG (and therefore of constitutive activation) of any receptor system depends upon how well the receptor forms the active state (value of L) and the relative ratio of receptor to G-protein. Figure 4-13 shows the level of spontaneously formed R_aG for a given receptor (with characteristic value of L). As can be seen from the curve relating receptor density to spontaneous activity, an increase in the receptor/G-protein ratio results in a constitutively activated system. At low receptor levels, no basal activity is observed and drugs produce either no response or a positive response (quiescent system, see Fig 4-13). At higher receptor levels, constitutive activity results. Such systems have a potential to screen for ligands because, theoretically, any chemical that interacts with the receptor will modify the microscopic equilibria between receptor states and alter the basal (but unstable) elevated level of R_aG. Hence, any chemical disruption of the unstable equilibria established in a constitutively active system will be detected. This detection of ligand-receptor interaction can be used as a screening tool in the search for new drugs. Ligands that bind differentially to the receptor array could either decrease or increase constitutive receptor activity (see Fig 4-13).

A *second* application of genetically controlled receptor systems is *to detect drugs that actively disrupt spontaneously coupled receptors.* Such drugs have negative efficacy and are referred to as *inverse agonists*. The therapeutic impact of inverse agonists is as yet unknown, but they have the potential to quiet

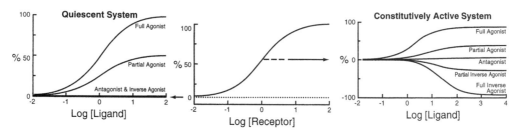

FIGURE 4-13. *The effects of constitutive receptor activity on drug-response profiles. The interdependence of receptor density ([R]) and G-protein concentration ([G]) on the amount of spontaneously active receptor/G-protein complex produced in a receptor system is shown in the middle panel. For a set amount of G-protein, increases in receptor levels lead to constitutive spontaneous response. The observed responses are to different types of drugs in systems with and without (quiescent) constitutive activity. Inverse agonists and antagonists are indistinguishable in quiescent systems, whereas they produce different effects in constitutively active systems.*

spontaneously active pathologic foci such as areas of dopamine receptor overexpression found in certain brain areas in patients with schizophrenia.

A *third* application of genetically modified receptor systems is the *control of receptor/G-protein pairs*. It is known that receptors are promiscuous with respect to the G-proteins with which they interact. Thus, one activated receptor may couple to two or more G-proteins in the membrane in response to activation by an agonist. It is not clear whether all agonists promote the production of a single activated state. Rather there is evidence that multiple activated states for receptors may exist. Therefore, the question arises; Do different agonists promote different spectra of activation states leading to differential activation of G-proteins? There is evidence that some agonists traffic stimulus to different G-protein pathways. This question may be extremely important in the design of specific agonists for therapy. For example, if the therapeutic effects of an agonist depend on one G-protein pathway and the side effects depend on another, theoretically it would be possible to eliminate the side effects by designing a similar agonist that traffics only to the beneficial pathway. Genetic engineering of receptor systems allows for the creation of cellular host systems with biased G-protein populations. The testing of agonists in such systems theoretically allows for the detection of agonist stimulus trafficking and the detection of more selective agonism. Figure 4-14 shows a schematic repre-

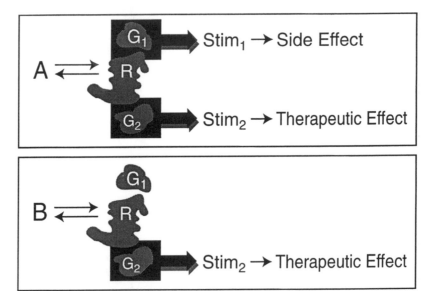

FIGURE 4-14. *Agonist trafficking of receptor stimulus. Agonist A produces an active state (or range of active states) that promiscuously activate(s) two G-proteins, giving rise to a useful effect and an unwanted side effect. Agonist B is more selective and produces a receptor active state that activates only the useful pathway. Selected genetically engineered assays are capable of distinguishing among these different profiles of agonism.*

sentation of stimulus trafficking and how it could affect therapeutic utility of an agonist.

4.6.2 Random Saturation Mutagenesis

As noted previously, the fact that receptors can exist in different tertiary conformational states and that some of these states are constitutively active has practical application in the screening of new drug entities. There also is considerable evidence that specific portions of the third intracellular loop of seven-transmembrane receptors activate G-proteins and that the inactive form of the receptor precludes access to this region (Fig 4-15). In contrast, the active form of the receptor exposes the critical region for G-protein activation. There is evidence that point mutations in receptors produce aberrant conformations that abstract the inactive state and, in fact, are predisposed to form

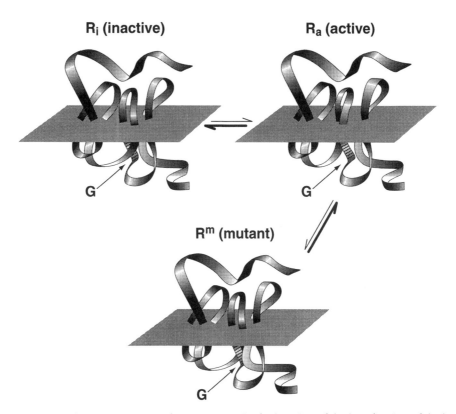

FIGURE 4-15. *Cartoons of a seven-transmembrane receptor in the inactivated (R_i) and activated (R_a) form. It is believed that a portion of the third intracellular loop (designated by horizontal bars) is essential in activating G-proteins and that this region of the receptor is hidden in the inactive form receptor and exposed in the active form. The receptor mutant R^m, by nature of its altered amino acid composition, more easily forms the active state, and thus systems possessing this mutant receptor are constitutively activated.*

the active state. These mutations often are constitutively active and thus are valuable in drug screening.

A prerequisite to the use of site-directed mutagenesis is prior knowledge of which region of the receptor is critical for G-protein coupling. However, an alternative method is to create a random library of cDNA that is mutated in the general region of G-protein coupling and to amplify the cDNA through PCR and screen for the constitutive active receptor. This technique, known as *random saturation mutagenesis*, introduces amino acid mutations in a region of the receptor without bias. The ability to detect constitutive activity (e.g., through reporter assays, *vide infra*) allows selection of the constitutive receptor. The cDNA then can be amplified through PCR and the receptor sequenced to determine the sequence of the mutant receptor.

4.7 SYNOPSIS

The following ideas were presented in this chapter:

- Receptor systems can be created by inserting human receptors into surrogate cell systems, thereby circumventing the shortcomings of using animal tissue.

- The gene for a particular receptor can be cloned leading to numerous copies of the gene in a form that can be manipulated.

- Either genomic or cDNA libraries can be constructed, and the passenger DNA pieces can be introduced into vectors. These can be made to replicate in bacterial cells. The clone of interest can be selected and amplified.

- Genes can be transfected into mammalian cells to create receptor testing systems. These systems can be temporary (transient transfection) or permanent (stable transfections).

- Genes for unknown products can be cloned and the product tested for function or presence (expression cloning). This can produce enough material to be characterized.

- The genetic code for protein products (i.e., receptors) can be used to determine receptor amino acid sequence. Alternatively, use of homologous sequences between receptors allows probing of gene libraries to detect related receptors of different structure.

- The polymerase chain reaction allows amplification of a single gene. This can be used to detect receptor genes and mutant receptor gene in tissues.

■ Genetic engineering can be used to custom-construct receptor systems for better screening of drugs and detection of weak drug activities.

FURTHER READING

Brown TA. Gene cloning, 2nd ed. London: Chapman and Hall, 1990.

Burstein ES, Spalding TA, Hill-Eubanks D, Brann MR. Structure-function of muscarinic receptor coupling to G-proteins. J Biol Chem 1995;270:3141–3146.

Darnell J, Lodish H, Baltimore D. Molecular cell biology, 2nd ed., New York: Freeman, 1990.

Davis L, Kuehl M, Battey J. Basic methods in molecular biology, 2nd ed. Norwalk, CT: Appleton and Lange, 1994.

Watson JD, Gilman M, Witkowski J, Zoller M. Recombinant DNA, 2nd ed. New York: Freeman, 1992.

Concentrations of Drugs in Tissues

5.1 Introduction

5.2 The Effects of Receptor Binding on Drug Concentration

5.3 Drug Adsorption to Protein and Surfaces

5.4 Biologic Degradation of Drugs in Living Tissues

5.5 Drug Diffusion in Tissues

5.6 Intracellular or Restricted-Access Compartments

5.7 Release of Endogenous Substances in Tissues

5.8 Synopsis

T HIS CHAPTER considers the only known independent variable in pharmacologic research from which all other parameters are derived, namely the concentration of drug at the biologic receptor. It follows, therefore, that the veracity of this quantity is paramount in pharmacologic research. There are mechanisms in biologic tissues that can produce differences between the amount of drug added to the system by the researcher and the actual amount producing the biologic response. These mechanisms include the binding of the drug to the receptor (section 5.2), adsorption to surfaces (section 5.3), and degradation by tissue uptake and enzyme systems (section 5.4). The process of drug removal from the receptor compartment depends on the process of diffusion in tissues (section 5.5) as receptors respond to a flux of concentration in the medium. This is exacerbated in restricted-access compartments such as the cytosol of the cell (section 5.6). A further complication can be seen with the release of endogenous biologically active substances from receptor systems (section 5.7). These ideas are reviewed in the chapter synopsis (section 5.8).

5.1 INTRODUCTION

Two tacit assumptions are made in all biologic experiments with drugs. The first is that the biologic tissue does not change the concentration of drug in the receptor compartment (i.e., the concentration of drug in the medium is infinite with respect to receptor uptake). The second is that the concentration of drug added to the medium bathing the biologic system is the same as that present in the receptor compartment (i.e., equal to that producing the drug response). It is worth challenging both of these assumptions in drug studies on biologic systems.

5.2 THE EFFECTS OF RECEPTOR BINDING ON DRUG CONCENTRATION

Most models of drug-receptor interaction are constructed under the assumption that the concentration of drug in the receptor compartment is not changed by the act of binding to the receptors (i.e., that there is an excess of drug bathing the surface of the cells containing the receptors). This assumption usually is valid in that the number of receptors activated by drugs most often is very small compared to the volume in bathing the tissue. Thus, under these circumstances, the fraction of drug bound to the receptor is very small compared to the total amount of drug in the medium. However, there are some circumstances in which this assumption is not valid, and it is worth examining the consequences of conditions in which this is the case. When this occurs, the concentration of drug free to bind to receptors (denoted $[A_{free}]$) is given by the subtractive product of the total concentration of drug ($[A_{total}]$) minus the concentration bound to receptor (which is equal to the concentration of drug-receptor complex $[A \cdot R]$). This changes the relationship between the concentration of drug in the receptor compartment and the amount of drug-receptor complex (as given by the Langmuir adsorption isotherm)(1). Thus, using $[A_{free}]$, the Langmuir adsorption isotherm can be rewritten as follows:

$$[A \cdot R] = \frac{([A_{total}] - [A \cdot R])[R_t]}{([A_{total}] - [A \cdot R]) + K_A} \qquad [5.1]$$

One solution for Equation 5.1 is the quadratic root:

$$[A \cdot R] = \frac{([A_t] + K_A + [R_t])}{2} + \left[\frac{(-[A_t] - K_A - [R_t])^2 - 4[A_t][R_t]}{4}\right]^{1/2} \qquad [5.2]$$

From Equation 5.2 it can be seen that the concentration of drug-receptor complex (and hence, the degree of cellular activation by the drug) can be limited by the amount of drug bound to the receptor (i.e., if $[R_t]>>[A_t]$) then $[A \cdot R]$ $[A_t]$: That is, the amount of drug-receptor complex formed is limited by the amount of drug added to the medium and not by mass action. This can be shown by the curvature in the relationship between the size of the receptor pool (quantified as a fraction of K_A, $[R_t]/[K_A]$) and the expected drug-receptor occupancy. If the drug concentration were infinite, then the relationship between $[R_t]/[K_A]$ and receptor occupancy would be a straight line (Fig 5-1). However, if the size of the receptor pool becomes large enough to deplete the pool of free drug, then the receptor occupancy by that drug eventually will decrease until the free concentration is zero and there is no further drug available to form $[A \cdot R]$. This is the horizontal region of the curve shown in Figure 5-1. Clearly, for the Langmuir adsorption isotherm to function as a realistic model for drug binding, the conditions must ensure that the concentration of drug is not affected by the amount of binding to receptors (i.e., that $[R_t]$ is kept low relative to the concentrations of drug used; the linear portion of the curve in Fig 5-1). This is a practical consideration in radioligand-binding studies in which the strength of signal can be increased by increasing the amount of cell membrane in the assay (i.e., increasing the number of receptors). Under these circumstances, if a poor binding signal is obtained from a given concentration of receptor-containing membrane, then the amount of tissue can be increased to strengthen the signal. The limitation, however, on this approach is that the large amount of receptor needed to generate the

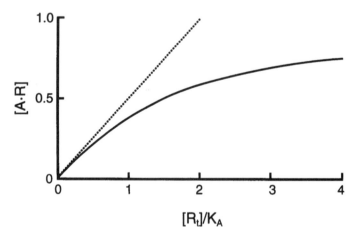

FIGURE 5-1. *The amount of drug-receptor complex ($[A \cdot R]$) formed for a concentration of drug equal to the K_A value under conditions of increasing receptor number ($[R_t]$ normalized by division by K_A). At low receptor concentrations the relationship between $[A \cdot R]$ and $[R_t]$ is linear (i.e., there is excess drug to bind to the receptor as needed). However, at higher receptor concentrations, the binding of the drug depletes the pool of drug left to bind and the relationship is no longer linear. At receptor concentrations greater than 4, the drug is bound completely, and an increase in receptor beyond this point results in no further formation of drug-receptor complex.*

signal may bind an appreciable fraction of the radiolabeled ligand, making the standard kinetic models of drug receptors inaccurate.

5.3 DRUG ADSORPTION TO PROTEIN AND SURFACES

Drugs are designed to interact with receptors in that they have stereochemistry and electrochemical characteristics that allow them to bind closely with complementary structures. These structures can be undesirable as well and as such can serve as sinks into which the drug can accumulate, to the detriment of fruitful receptor binding. A most common sink is protein in the bloodstream when drugs are given in vivo. In experimental studies designed to determine drug potency, surfaces can adsorb drugs and deplete the concentration in the bathing medium and, subsequently, in the receptor compartment. Under these circumstances, the concentration of drug added by the experimenter and that present in the medium are different. In pharmacologic terms, such effects are a hindrance to the quantification of drug-receptor responses. This is because all measures of the dependent variables that quantify drug activity are predicated on the accurate value for the independent variable—namely, the concentration of drug believed to be present at the receptor. If this latter value is incorrect, so too will be all resulting calculations. Therefore, it is of paramount importance that the correct magnitude of the independent parameter in pharmacologic experiments be known.

One way to examine the effects of drug adsorption is to model the adsorption surface (or amount of drug-binding protein) as a "concentration" of drug binding sites (denoted $[B]$) with a macro-affinity constant K'_B. In this case, this is the averaged affinity for what probably is a large number of heterogeneous sites, all with different sensitivities to drug binding. Under these circumstances, the drug bound to the surface ($[A_{bound}]$) as a fraction of the total drug concentration ($[A_{total}]$) is given by:

$$\frac{[A_{bound}]}{[A_{total}]} = \left[1 + \frac{K'_B}{[B]} + \frac{[A]}{[B]}\right]^{-1} \qquad [5.3]$$

This equation quantifies what would be expected intuitively—namely that if the concentration of adsorption sites is low (small $[B]$) or if the affinity of the drug for the adsorption sites is low (high K'_B), then the ratio $[A_{bound}]/[A_{total}]$ will be small (i.e., little drug will be adsorbed). Also equation 5.3 indicates that adsorption of drugs into a sink theoretically is saturable and that extremely high concentrations of A can reduce the bound ratio to insignificant proportions ($[A] \gg [B]$). In practical terms, however, if $[B]$ is very large, as in the surface of a reaction tube or cell culture dish, the adsorption effect may behave as if it were unsaturable.

The fact that the degree of adsorption depends on both [B] and [A], can be seen from the equation describing the occupancy of a receptor population by drug [A] in the presence of a conflicting population of adsorption sites at concentration [B]:

$$\rho = \left[1 + \frac{K_A([B] + K'_B + [A])}{[A]\,(K'_B + [A])} \right]^{-1} \qquad [5.4]$$

where K_A is the equilibrium dissociation constant for the drug-receptor complex. This equation predicts that, given a high enough concentration of [A], the effects of a given concentration of adsorption sites can be overcome and the original maximal response to A, obtained in the absence of [B], will be achieved. The effects of drug adsorption on the dose-response curves to drug A are shown in Figure 5-2. Two cases are shown. In figure 5-2A, the affinity of the drug for the adsorption is greater than that for the receptor ($K'_B < K_A$). Under these circumstances, low doses of drug will be adsorbed to a greater extent than high doses and the slope of the dose-response curve will change

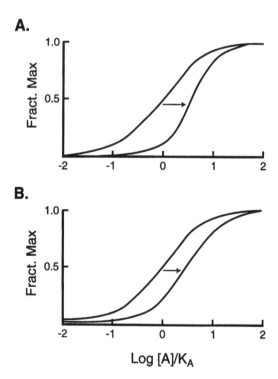

FIGURE 5-2. *Adsorption of drug to inert surfaces. A. When the affinity of the drug for the surface is greater than that for the receptor, then a nonparallel shift to the right occurs. B. When the affinity of the drug for the receptor is greater than that for the surface, a parallel shift to the right is observed.*

(i.e., the slope will increase with increasing doses of drug). Observance of such changes in slope is one method of detecting appreciable adsorption of drugs. Figure 5-2B shows another scenario whereby the affinity of the drug for the receptor is greater than for the adsorption sites (K'_B K_A). Under these circumstances, parallel shifts of the dose-response curve will be produced by adsorption.

Serious obfuscations in the relative potency of drugs can be produced by adsorption of drug to nonreceptor sites. Experiments with radioactive tracer drugs show that surfaces can bind 400 to 500 times greater concentrations than receptors. If undetected, these effects will be interpreted as differences in primary drug activity. Figure 5-3 shows a simulation comparing two drugs that are *equiactive* for biologic receptors but that differ in sensitivity to adsorption to the surface of the culture dish housing the cells (K'_B for drug *A* is 1000 times K'_B for Drug *B*). The observed relative potency of these drugs differs by a factor of 10, an artifact of adsorption. It is essential to recognize such effects because they probably will differ under different experimental conditions and certainly in vivo in the therapeutic environment.

Though adsorption is a problem in pharmacologic experiments bent on the quantification of drug activity, the uptake and biologic degradation of drugs also are very important. The effects of enzymatic destruction of drugs

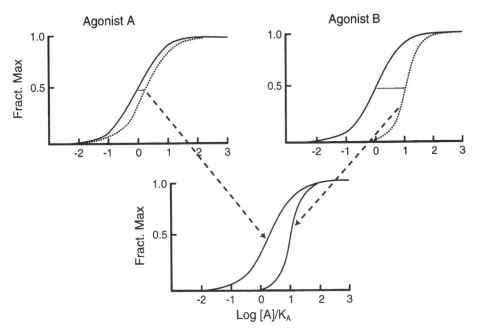

FIGURE 5-3. *Two equiactive agonists are adsorbed to surfaces to varying degrees. The result is a difference in the observed potencies of the two agonists that is completely the result of the differential sensitivity of the agonists to adsorption.*

or active transport of drugs away from the receptor compartment are qualitatively similar to the effectes of adsorption to an inert surface.

5.4 BIOLOGIC DEGRADATION OF DRUGS IN LIVING TISSUES

Biologic tissues are very responsive to endogenous chemicals (hormones, neurotransmitters), and the temporal and spatial control of responses to these chemicals often is achieved through avid removal and degradation mechanisms. The added ability of tissues to remove the agonist by biochemical means (or to cease to remove the chemical in the case of saturating concentrations) results in another mode of function control. For example, a powerful removal mechanism for the neurotransmitter norepinephrine is neuronal uptake and a spatial pattern of concentration distribution can be achieved by the overlay of neural norepinephrine uptake sites on tissues containing neurons possessing this mechanism.

In general, the spatial relationships between the sites of drug removal and the receptors are important. Thus, a removal process that acts as a barrier between the drug and the receptor compartment (Fig 5-4A) could have a profound effect on the concentrations of drug reaching the receptors. In contrast, if the sites of drug removal are parallel to the receptors (Fig 5-4B) or reside beyond the receptors (Fig 5-4C), then progressively less effect on receptor concentrations of drug may be observed. However, in all these cases, it should be noted that the receptors respond to a *flux* of drug concentrations (i.e., a flow from the bathing medium); therefore, the avidity of drug removal also depends on the rate of delivery of the drug to the receptor compartment (*vide infra*).

Under these circumstances, only a portion of the drug added to the medium will, in fact, reach the receptors. Because the concentration of drug added to the medium is known by the experimenter and it is assumed to be present in the receptor compartment, then a dissimulation will occur in that the observed location of the dose-response curve for the drug will not reflect the true potency of the drug (Fig 5-5).

It is useful to examine a simple model of drug removal in the receptor compartment as a focus for discussion of the factors involved. In general, it can be said that receptors are subjected to a flux of drug consisting of entry into the receptor compartment, usually by bulk diffusion (or the circulatory system), and removal by either an active process or diffusion. An active removal system such as uptake or an enzymatic degradation can be described by saturable Michaelis-Menten kinetics, whereby the rate of removal (J) is governed by the following equation:

$$J = \frac{[A_i]J_{max}}{[A_i] + K_m} \qquad [5.5]$$

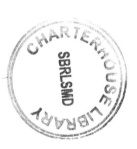

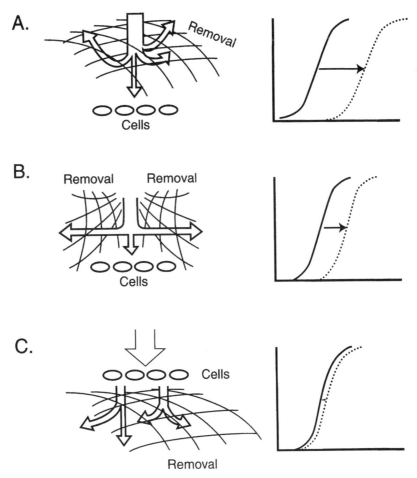

FIGURE 5-4. *Effects of geometric relationships between drug removal and receptors on observed potency. A. The site of drug removal lies in the path of drug diffusion to the receptors. This results in a large deficit of agonist and a resulting large shift to the right of the observed dose-response curve. B. The site of removal is parallel to the receptors. The effects on the agonist dose-response curve are reduced compared to the situation in A. C. The site of removal is beyond the receptor compartment. The effects on the agonist dose-response curve are minimal.*

where K_m refers to the saturable Michaelis-Menten constant for the removal mechanism, A_i is the relative concentration of drug A in the receptor compartment and J_{max} is the maximal capacity of the removal mechanism.

A general equation to describe this interplay of processes can be derived (1):

$$[A_i] = \frac{-(K_m + (J_{max}\ V/k_{in}S) - [A_0])}{2} + \left[\frac{(K_m + (J_{max}\ V/k_{in}S) - [A_0])^2}{4} + K_m[A_0] \right]^{1/2} \qquad [5.6]$$

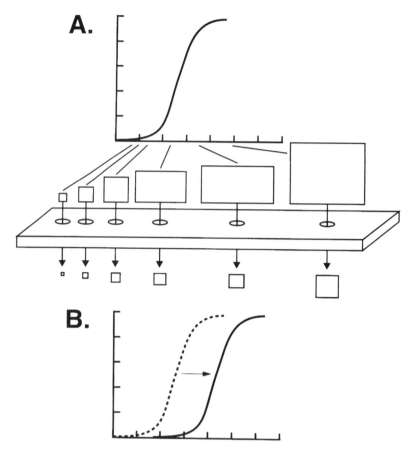

FIGURE 5-5. *The effects of an agonist removal mechanism on the observed agonist dose-response curve. A. The true agonist potency. B. The observed potency due to the diminution of agonist concentration produced by the agonist removal mechanism. The dotted line shows the true curve, the solid line the observed curve.*

where the relative concentrations of drug A in the receptor compartment and out of it are given by $[A_i]$ and $[A_0]$, respectively; V and S are the volume and surface area of the tissue or cell mass, respectively, and k_{in} refers to the diffusion rate constant for the drug.

In general, Equation 5.6 indicates the following about the differences between drug concentration in the receptor compartment and in the outer medium bathing the tissue or cells:

1. Reduced by a high diffusion rate into the compartment (high k_{in})

2. Increased by a high capacity for removal (J_{max})

3. Increased by a large-volume tissue mass but reduced by a large surface area to the tissue (cell) mass

4. Reduced by concentrations of drug that saturate the removal system ($[A_0] \gg K_m$)

The sensitization of tissues by inhibition of removal mechanisms can be quantified by the following equation:

$$\varphi = \frac{\psi \, (1 + [I]/K_I)}{\psi + [I]/K_I} \qquad [5.7]$$

where $[I]$ is the concentration of inhibitor of the removal process, K_I is the equilibrium dissociation constant of the inhibitor/removal-site complex, ψ is maximal sensitization possible after complete inhibition of the removal process, and φ is the sensitization in the presence of the given concentration of inhibitor for the removal process (Fig 5-6A). It can be seen that a series of sensitizations can be used to furnish an estimate of the potency of the inhibitor (the K_I for the site of removal) through a logarithmic metameter of Equation 5.7 (2):

$$\text{Log} \left[\frac{\psi(\varphi - 1)}{\psi - \varphi} \right] = \text{Log} \, [I] - \text{Log} \, K_I \qquad [5.8]$$

Thus, a collection of φ values for a corresponding array of $[I]$ concentrations according to Equation 5.8 should yield a straight line with a slope of unity and an intercept of pK_I ($-\text{Log} \, K_I$); see Figure 5-6B.

A plot of the fractional sensitization (φ/ψ) for any given concentration of inhibitor for removal shows that the larger the maximal effect of the removal process (the higher the sensitivity of the drug to removal; large ψ), the more difficult it is to negate the effects of removal (the higher the concentration of $[I]$ needed to produce full sensitization; Figure 5-7). The complete negation of a removal process for a drug in a tissue may require a concentration of inhibitor considerably greater than the K_I. As can be seen from Figure 5-7, if the removal process produces a 100-fold difference between the concentration of drug added to the medium and that in the receptor compartment, then a concentration of inhibitor 100 times the K_I would be required to produce a 50% inhibition of the process. From Equation 5.7 it can be seen that to achieve near-complete (90%) inhibition of drug removal from a system that produces a 100-fold decrease in the receptor compartment concentration of drug, then 890 times the K_I would be needed. Unless the potency of the blocker for the uptake process is very high, the concentrations of inhibitor required for complete inhibition of drug removal may exceed practical limits of selectivity and secondary drug effects may be encountered. However, the absolute potencies of drugs usually are not relevant to the drug and receptor classification process but rather the relative potency of different drugs is what is required. This is fortunate from the point of view of negating

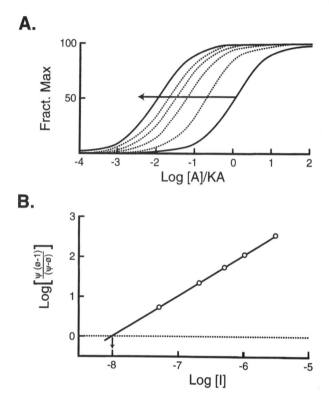

FIGURE 5-6. *The effects of inhibition of agonist removal mechanisms on the location of agonist dose-response curves. A. The dose-response curve furthest to the right is observed in the absence of removal mechanism inhibition (i.e., the full effects of the removal mechanism are operative). With increasing addition of inhibitor for agonist removal, the dose-response curve shifts to the left (i.e., more of the added agonist reaches the receptor compartment). At maximal inhibition of the removal mechanism, a maximal sensitization of the agonist response is achieved (i.e., the curve can no longer be shifted to the left). B. The sensitizations produced by inhibition of the removal mechanism (at given concentrations of uptake inhibitor [I]) are plotted according to Equation 5.8. The resulting regression is linear, with an intercept that is an estimate of the − Log K of the removal process inhibitor for the site of removal.*

the removal of drug from the receptor compartment, as the negation of removal effects on the relative potency of two drugs is more sensitive to inhibitors than is the absolute potency of either one of the drugs. This is shown in Figure 5-8, where two drugs are compared, one removed from the receptor compartment by a factor of 100 and one removed by a factor of 10. In the absence of the removal mechanism, both drugs are equipotent. In the presence of the active removal process, the drugs appear to differ in potency by a factor of ten (i.e., the removal process produces an apparent difference in potency of 10). The abscissal axis of Figure 5-8 shows the concentrations

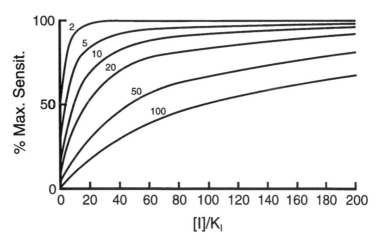

FIGURE 5-7. *The sensitization to an agonist produced by inhibition of a removal process, expressed as a fraction of the maximal sensitization in the system, as a function of the concentration of inhibitor for the removal process. Note that more uptake blocker is required to negate the effects of removal in systems in which the maximal effects of the removal are largest: That is, whereas a value of $[I]/K_I = 20$ is sufficient to cancel the effects of removal in a system in which the maximal sensitization is 2, this value produces only a 25% inhibition for a system in which the maximal sensitization is 50.*

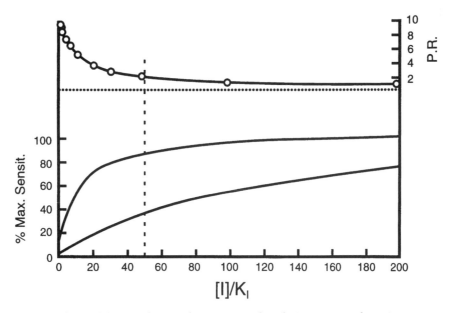

FIGURE 5-8. *The effects of the inhibition of removal processes on the relative potency of agonists. Bottom curves show sensitization to two agonists. One is severely affected by removal ($\psi = 100$) and one is less affected ($\psi = 10$). At a concentration of removal inhibitor of 50, it can be seen that the sensitization of the system to the two agonists is at best partial. However, as shown on the top curve, the relative potency of the two drugs (they are equipotent in the absence of agonist removal) approaches the true value: That is, less uptake blocker is required to correct the effects of removal on relative potency than is required for absolute potency.*

of inhibitor of the drug removal process. It can be seen that at a concentration of $[I]/K_I = 50$, the relative sensitization of the tissue to both agonists is, at best, partial but that the relative potency of the two drugs has already approached 2.28, an acceptable approximation of the true value of unity. Thus, while the absolute potency of either drug is incorrect with this concentration of inhibitor in the medium, the relative potency is nearly correct. As a general rule, the relative potency of drugs removed from the receptor compartment by an active process is more amenable to correction by uptake inhibition than is the absolute potency.

Differences between the known added concentration of drug to the biologic preparation and the actual concentration in the receptor compartment (changed by either removal by an active process or adsorption to a surface or other structure in the preparation) can be very dissimulating in that they produce artifacts of potency estimates that then are translated to artifacts in affinity and efficacy of drugs. Therefore, it is of practical importance to detect and negate these processes in receptor pharmacology. Detection can be difficult, especially in the absence of other drugs to block the obfuscating process. In general, changes in the slope of dose-response curves can suggest the presence of a saturable removal process. The addition of substances that can counter adsorption to surfaces (i.e., lysine, arginine, bovine serum albumin, choline, polylysine, polyethylineimine) also can be used to render surfaces inert to adsorption of some drugs. A very powerful method of detecting removal processes is by the observation of the slope of Schild regressions (see Chapter 8).

5.5 DRUG DIFFUSION IN TISSUES

As discussed earlier, the effect of a removal or adsorption process on the concentration of drug accessible to the receptors depends directly on the rate of delivery of the drug to the receptor compartment. If this rate of delivery is slow, a fairly weak removal process *still* could seriously diminish the concentration of drug reaching the receptors. Alternatively, if the rate of delivery is rapid, then the weak removal process will be inconsequential. The delivery of a drug to the receptor compartment is by bulk diffusion which can be affected by the unstirred water layer surrounding the biologic preparation, the viscosity of the medium, and the tortuosity of the tissue structure. Usually, viscosity is not an appreciable factor as biologic tissues always are in aqueous-based media, but added protein (i.e. bovine serum albumin, plasma) and the latticelike microstructures of water surrounding receptor may reduce drug mobility near drug receptors (3).

The first obstruction to free diffusion that a drug will encounter is the unstirred water layer surrounding the biologic structure. Within this layer, diffusion is slowed appreciably; therefore, its thickness is a variable that can affect general drug access to the tissue. The half-time for diffusion through an unstirred water layer of thickness δ can be approximated by the following equation (4):

$$t_{1/2} = 0.38\delta^2/D \qquad [5.9]$$

where D is the diffusion coefficient in the medium (the factor sensitive to viscosity, hydration shells, etc.). Stirring can reduce the thickness of the unstirred water layer and subsequently increase the rate of access of the drug to the tissue. Figure 5.9 shows the effect of δ thickness on $t_{1/2}$ and the approximated effect of no stirring and introducing a stirring motion of 1200 rpm.

A second factor for drug access to receptors is tortuosity which characterizes the ease with which the drug can diffuse within the structure of the tissue to access the extracellular space. The diffusion of drug within the tissue (denoted D') is given by the diffusion in the free medium (D) divided by the square of the tortuosity factor:

$$D' = D/\lambda^2 \qquad [5.10]$$

Tortuosity is a tissue-specific factor and should be constant for a given biologic preparation, although in the case of cell culture monolayers, the degree of cellular interconnection might change from preparation to preparation and be variable between experiments. The rate of penetration of a drug into the receptor compartment of a tissue (denoted k_{in}) is given by the following relationship:

$$k_{in} = \frac{\kappa_{tissue}}{1 + (\kappa_{tissue}(\delta/D))} \qquad [5.11]$$

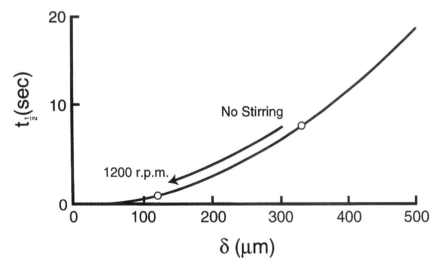

FIGURE 5-9. *The half-time ($t_{1/2}$) for diffusion from the medium to the tissue surface through the unstirred water layer. Note the decrease in this half-time with stirring at 1200 rpm.*

where κ_{tissue} is a permeation constant characterizing the tortuosity of the preparation, δ is the unstirred water layer, and D is the free diffusion coefficient in the medium. It can be seen from this equation that the diffusion within the tissue will be lower than in the medium if either the permeation factor κ_{tissue} is low (high tortuosity) or there is a thick, unstirred water layer surrounding the preparation (Fig 5-10).

In general, *in the absence of major removal mechanisms for drugs in tissues* (i.e., degradative enzymes, uptake processes, adsorption sites), the rate of diffusion in tissues is not a relevant experimental factor because it affects only the rate of approach to equilibrium. Because all estimates of drug activity are made at equilibrium (or as near as possible to equilibrium), diffusion cannot affect measures of drug potency or biologic activity. The one possible exception to this condition is if the drug is chemically unstable. Under these circumstances, the rate of presentation to the receptor compartment could affect the magnitude of biologic response.

The relationship between the drug response of a biologic tissue and the concentration of drug required to elicit that response depends on a number of factors, some related to the drug (affinity and efficacy) and some related to the tissue (the receptor density, efficiency of stimulus-response coupling). This latter factor reflects the efficiency of the coupling between the receptors as responding units and the total response capability of the tissue. An impor-

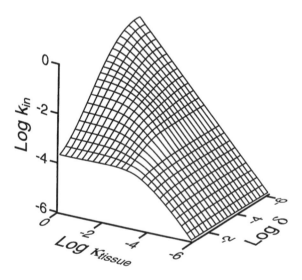

FIGURE 5-10. *The relationship between the permeation constant (κ, log scale) and thickness of the unstirred water layer (δ, log scale) on the rate constant for entry of a drug into a tissue array. Note that for thick, unstirred water layers or low permeation constants, the rate of entry of the drug is slow (low k_{in}).*

tant facet of this efficiency is the mechanical and electrical coupling of cells within tissues.

Many tissues have tight junctions that facilitate electrical cell-to-cell coupling. Under these circumstances, not all of the tissue need be activated by the drug for the complete syncytial tissue response to be elicited. The activation of a collection of cells can be viewed as the triggering of an array of responding units of varying threshold. The resulting signals take on a Boltzmann distribution, with the most sensitive cells firing at low drug concentrations and increasing recruitment of firing cells with increasing drug concentrations (Fig 5-11A). The cumulative signal from this distribution provides the drug's familiar sigmoidal dose-response curve (Fig 5-11B). If some of the cells are coupled to others such that when they fire the coupled cells also will fire, then the distribution of the collective firing of the complete population will be more focused (see Fig 5-11A, distribution 2). Further coupling will focus the distribution further (Fig 5-11A, distribution 3); the resulting dose-response curves for these preparations will be correspondingly more steep. This illustrates the futility of using the shape of the functional dose-response curve from a biologic preparation to determine the stoichiometry or mechanism of drug-receptor interaction. In all cases,

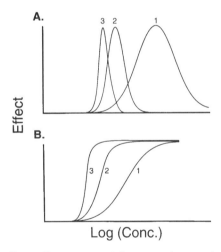

FIGURE 5-11. *The effects of cell-to-cell coupling on syncytial response in organized tissue arrays. A. The sensitivity of an array of cells to a drug, described as a distribution. For distribution 1, the drug must activate each of the cells individually. The system depicted by distribution 2 has some cell-to-cell coupling (i.e., the activation of one cell leads automatically to the activation of a number of other cells through electrical coupling). Distribution 3 is for a highly coupled system wherein the activation of only a few cells leads to the activation of most of the other cells. B. The predicted dose-response curves for the three systems shown in A. Note that as cell-to-cell coupling increases, the system becomes more sensitive and the curves become steeper.*

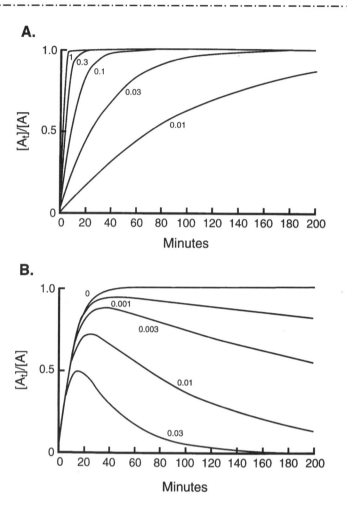

FIGURE 5-12. *The diffusion of drugs into restricted compartments. A. The fractional entry of drugs into the receptor compartment with time, for systems of differing rate constants for delivery (Q/V= 1, 0.3, 0.1, 0.01). B. Diffusion of a drug with a rate of entry Q/V= 0.1 into compartments of varying rates of removal (k_{out} = 0, 0.001, 0.003, 0.01, 0.03). Note that when removal is appreciable, the peak concentration for the drug falls short of the equilibrium concentration for a system where there is no removal.*

the stimulus-response mechanisms of the biologic tissue control the shape of the curve, irrespective of the kinetics of the interaction between the drug and the receptor.

5.6 INTRACELLULAR OR RESTRICTED-ACCESS COMPARTMENTS

Many drugs must gain entry into the cell to find their respective receptors and elicit response. The plasma membrane can be a formidable barrier to free access of drugs, but the drugs can get around this barrier in a variety of ways, from passive diffusion through the lipid membrane, to active transport, a channel, or endocytosis. In terms of drug-receptor classification, these mechanisms can lead effectively to a highly restricted diffusion. The concentration of drug in a restricted compartment at time t [A_t] is given by Equation 5.12 (5):

$$[A_t] = [A](1 - e^{-(Q/V)t})$$ [5.12]

where Q is the rate of drug delivery to the restricted compartment and V is the volume of the compartment. It is assumed that the concentration of the drug in the extracellular compartment rises instantaneously to a value [A]. It can be seen from Figure 5-12A that if the volume of the intracellular compartment is large or the rate of delivery is slow, the rise of concentration of drug in the cell will be correspondingly slow.

A further complication arises if the drug is degraded in the cell cytosol. Under these circumstances, the amount of drug available to produce effect inside the cell is a flux controlled by the rate of entry into the cell and the rate of degradation in the cell. The concentration of drug in the cytosol with time is given by the following equation:

$$[A_t] = [A]\,(e^{-k_{out}t})\,(1 - e^{-(Q/V)t})$$ [5.13]

where the rate of degradation is approximated by a rate of outflow from the receptor compartment, denoted k_{out}. The concentrations of such a drug with time under conditions of varying rates of cytosolic degradation are shown in Figure 5-12B. Two features of this figure are the fact that the amount of drug in the receptor compartment declines with time (i.e., a steady state is not observed unless k_{out} is very much lower than Q/V) and, depending on the relative magnitudes of k_{out} and Q/V, the peak concentration that would have been achieved in the absence of drug degradation may never be achieved in such a system (i.e., the maxima for the concentration time curves are below unity).

5.7 RELEASE OF ENDOGENOUS SUBSTANCES IN TISSUES

As well as being degraded in biologic systems, drugs can cause the release of endogenous biologically active substances in tissues; such drugs will be referred to as *indirect agonists*. It is important to know when this occurs so as not to ascribe the activity to the releasing drug. The potency of indirect agonists depends upon the usual tissue effects of stimulus-response processing and the efficacy and affinity (denoted K_A) of the released agonist as well

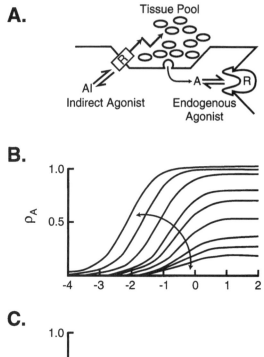

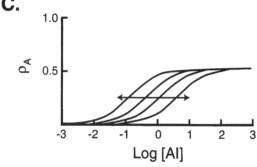

FIGURE 5-13. *The effects of an indirect agonist. A. Schematic diagram of an indirect agonist (AI) interacting with a recognition site R to affect the release of an endogenous agonist A from a tissue pool. The endogenous agonist interacts with the tissue receptor. B. The effects on the observed indirect agonist dose-response curve varying the effective pool size of endogenous agonist. Note that both the maximal asymptote and the location parameter of the dose-response changes. C. Effects of varying the affinity of the indirect agonist for the site of recognition for the indirect agonist for release. Changes in this parameter (K_{AI}) produce changes only in the location of the dose-response curve to the indirect agonist, not the maximal asymptote.*

as two additional factors. These are the size of the pool of endogenous agonist (accounted for by the factor θ, *vide infra*) and the affinity of the indirect agonist for the site of release (denoted K_{AI}). Assuming that the tissue response emanates from a released concentration of endogenous agonist (Fig 5-13A), the fractional occupancy of the receptors by this endogenous agonist ρ_{AI} can be expressed as a function of the concentration of indirect agonist (6):

$$\rho_{AI} = \left[1 + \frac{K_{AI}}{\theta} 1 + \frac{K_A}{[A]} \right]^{-1} \qquad [5.13]$$

where K_{AI} and K_A are the equilibrium dissociation constants for the indirect agonist and site of release and the released agonist and receptor respectively. An indirect agonist has basically two properties. The first is an affinity for the site of release; this is characterized by K_{AI}. The second property is the *efficacy* with which the drug causes release of the endogenous agonist. This drug property is expressed in various tissues in conjunction with a tissue factor—namely, the size of the pool of endogenous agonist to be released. Thus, the factor θ is a mixture of the ability of the indirect agonist to initiate release and the size of the releasable pool. Figure 5-13B shows the effects on the dose-response curve to an indirect agonist of varying θ. It can be seen that both the location of the curve and the maximal response attained vary with both the efficacy of the drug causing release and the size of the pool of endogenous agonist. In contrast, Figure 5-13C shows the effects on the dose-response curve to various indirect agonists of varying K_{AI}. Here it can be seen that the maximal response of the indirect agonist is not affected by changes in affinity for the site of release but only by the location of the dose-response curve.

5.8 SYNOPSIS

The following ideas were presented in this chapter:

- All receptor theory is based on the assumption that the concentration of drug in the receptor compartment is known and that the binding of drug to receptor does not change it.

- All experimental procedures should be carried out in a region where the relationship between receptor density and drug concentration is linear; this ensures that drug concentration is not affected by receptor binding.

- Drugs may adsorb to a large number of nonreceptor sites (protein, surfaces). This can cause a shift to the right of the dose-response curve (either parallel shift or an increase in the slope).

- Biologic tissues can degrade or otherwise remove drugs from the receptor compartment. Receptors react to a flux of drug coming out of the bathing medium by diffusion and out of the receptor compartment via active processes that can be modeled by Michaelis-Menten kinetics.

- In general, deficits of concentration near receptors are exacerbated by slow diffusion (high tissue structure, low surface-to-volume ratios, avid maximal removal mechanisms). The larger the effects of drug removal, the higher is the concentration of removal inhibitor required to negate them.

- Diffusion of drug into structured biologic tissues is hampered by the existence of unstirred water layers on the surface.

- Cell-to-cell coupling in tissues allows syncytial tissue response to occur with activation of only a fraction of the cells.

- Drug concentration may never reach the level in the extracellular space in highly restricted compartments (i.e., the cytosol) in which active degradation mechanisms are operative.

- Indirect agonists can cause release of endogenous agonists in tissues.

REFERENCES

1. Furchgott RF. The classification of adrenoceptors (adrenergic receptors). An evaluation from the standpoint of receptor theory. In: Blaschko H, Muscholl E, eds. Handbook of experimental pharmacology: catecholamines, vol. 33. Berlin: Spinger-Verlag, 1977: 283–335.
2. Kenakin TP, Beek D.The measurement of antagonist potency and the importance of selective inhibition of agonist removal processes. J Pharmacol Exp Ther 1981;219:112–120.
3. Crank J. The mathematics of diffusion (second edition). Oxford: Clarendon Press, 1975.
4. Cuthbert AW, Dunant Y. Diffusion of drugs through stationary water layers as the rate limiting process in their action on membrane receptors. Br J Pharmacol 1970;40:508–521.
5. Waud DR. On diffusion from a point source. J Pharmacol Exp Ther 1968;159:123–128.
6. Black JW, Jenkinson DH, Kenakin TP. Antagonism of an indirectly acting agonist: Block by propranolol and sotalol of the action of tyramine on rat heart. Eur J Pharmacol 1981;65:1–10.

FURTHER READING

Foster RW. The potentiation of responses to noradrenaline and isoprenaline in guinea pig isolated tracheal chain preparations by desipramine, cocaine, phentolamine, phenoxybenzamine, guanethidine, metanephrine, and cooling. Br J Pharmacol Chemother 1967;31:418–427.

Kenakin TP. A pharmacological method to estimate the pK_I of competitive inhibitors of agonist uptake processes in isolated tissues. Naunyn Schmiedeberg's Arch Pharmacol 1981;316:89–95.

Kenakin TP. On the importance of agonist concentration-gradients within isolated tissues. Increased maximal response of rat vasa deferentia to (-)-noradrenaline after blockade of neuronal uptake. J Pharm Pharmacol 1980;32:833–838.

Agonism and Stimulus-Response Mechanisms

THE ESSENCE OF pharmacology concerns the mechanisms of efficacy: How can a receptor protein repeatedly produce a change in a biologic system in response to chemical stimuli without a chemical reaction occurring between the two? Direct agonism (section 6.2) discusses the processes whereby agonists "isomerize" receptors and thus change their state. Some general principles by which cells process this receptor signal to produce physiologic response are reviewed in section 6.3. The measurement of the relative ability of different agonists to initiate response is vital to the classification of receptors and the discovery of new drugs. This can be done operationally with no required knowledge of molecular mechanism (section 6.4). Such molecular mechanisms have been postulated and are reviewed in section 6.5. The potentiation of endogenous substances as a mechanism of agonism is discussed in section 6.6. Finally, these ideas are reviewed in the chapter synopsis (section 6.7).

6.1 GENERAL MECHANISMS OF AGONISM

As described in Chapter 1, drugs can initiate biochemical processes or modify ongoing biochemical processes in cells. It should be noted that these effects can take the form of *stimulation* (i.e., an increase in the biologic readout) or *depression* of a system. *Response* thus is defined as a change, with no reference to increase or decrease. Biologic systems are extremely complex and are composed of numerous ongoing mechanisms that function at various levels of activity. Therefore, the initial activation of a target receptor can have far-reaching consequences to the biologic host. Moreover, activation of the same target in different hosts can lead to completely different physiologic responses. This is in keeping with the modular nature of biologic systems (i.e., different combinations of receptors and biochemical cascade systems; see Fig 1-3).

Drugs can produce cellular response in one of two ways—by *direct* or *indirect* agonism. Direct agonism involves a response emanating from the interaction of an agonist with a receptor with a resulting change in state of that receptor. This interaction can take the form of *initiation* or *inhibition* of a cellular process. *Indirect agonism* results from a drug affecting the action of an endogenous substance (i.e., a chemical that already is mediating a cellular process). This interaction can take the form of *potentiation* or *modulation*. A special case of indirect agonism also can be found in drugs that cause the release of an endogenous agonist, as discussed in Chapter 5.

The process of direct agonism is the result of the activation of a receptor by a drug with intrinsic efficacy. Some receptors can be constitutively active; that is, they produce response on their own in the absence of an agonist. Under these circumstances, some drugs actively reverse this activity (inverse agonists; see Chapter 1). The molecular mechanisms involved are identical to those that initiate response. Indirect agonism usually is allosteric in nature (see Chapter 1) in that a drug binds to a receptor at a site different from that used by an endogenous molecule involved in the cellular process and, by doing so, makes the existing biochemical reaction more efficient. A variant of this mechanism is one in which a drug blocks an ongoing endogenous process and negates the basal cellular activity that was present in the absence of the drug. This often is achieved by the blockade of an uptake or degradatory process.

In this chapter direct and indirect agonism are discussed separately. By far the more simple mechanism with which to determine drug and predict drug activity in humans is direct agonism. Indirect agonism is more complex in that the mechanisms by which a ligand causes potentiation, modulation of basal tone, or release of endogenous agonists does not involve intrinsic efficacy but rather results from ligand affinity to different binding sites. The expression of indirect agonism is extremely dependent on the host system and, in many cases, on the receptor environment in vivo.

6.2 DIRECT AGONISM

In general, direct agonism consists of two steps: the process of an agonist imparting the signal to the receptor to activate it and the process of the activated receptor transmitting the signal to the cellular machinery to induce cellular response. Conceptually, this transmission can be thought of in terms of a drug-induced change in the receptor—in effect, a receptor isomerization.

6.2.1 Receptor Isomerization

Operationally, receptors can be thought of as recognition sites for hormones, neurotransmitters, and other drugs. It is the unique property of the agonist—namely, intrinsic efficacy—that causes the receptor to impart physiologic signals to the host upon agonist binding. Thus, the reaction can be viewed as follows:

$$A + R \underset{k_{-1}}{\overset{k_{+1}}{\rightleftharpoons}} A \cdot R \underset{\alpha}{\overset{\beta}{\rightleftharpoons}} A \cdot R^* \qquad [6.1]$$

where R is the receptor in recognition mode and R^* is the receptor in active mode from which point it goes on to cause physiologic response. The binding of the drug A to the receptor is controlled by the forward rate constant k_{+1}, and the dissociation of the drug from the receptor is controlled by the back rate constant k_{-1}. The equilibrium dissociation constant for drug binding thus is given as k_{-1}/k_{+1} and is denoted as K_{eq}. The propensity for the bound receptor to go on to the active form R^* is driven by the forward rate constant β and the propensity for the activated receptor to return to the inactive form is driven by α. The process of conversion of receptor from R to R^* (by agonist from $A \cdot R$ to $A \cdot R^*$) is termed *receptor isomerization* (Fig 6-1). This can be considered a general mechanism of agonism, and the equations that control the formation of the isomerized species can generally be helpful in describing a great many drug interactions with different receptor types.

There are consequences to the location parameter of the dose-response curve due to receptor isomerization. Specifically, the K_{obs} for the production of response is not controlled numerically by the magnitude of K_{eq} or β/α but

Agonist Binding

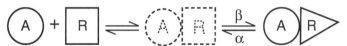

Receptor Isomerization

FIGURE 6-1. *The isomerization of receptors by agonists. Agonist A binds to the receptor and forms a complex AR, which transforms into a modified complex AR according to the forward and backward reaction rate, β and α, respectively. The transformation from the square receptor species to the triangular receptor species is termed isomerization. When this occurs, it drives the first binding reaction (A + R) forward.*

rather by an amalgam of the two constants. This is because, as for receptors in two states (see Chapter 4), the conversion of a receptor from AR to AR^* removes the R form from the equilibrium between $[A]$ and $[R]$ and therefore more AR must form to take its place. In this way, the reaction controlled by β/α drives the total reaction between $[A]$ and $[R]$ toward AR^*. The complete reaction should be viewed as follows:

$$A + R \underset{k_{-1}}{\overset{k_{+1}}{\rightleftharpoons}} A \cdot R \underset{\alpha}{\overset{\beta}{\rightleftharpoons}} A \cdot R^* \qquad [6.2]$$

with the K_{obs} [observed 50% effective dose (ED$_{50}$)] being dependent on K_{eq} and β/α. According to this scheme, the observed location parameter for the curve describing the complete process (K_{obs}) is given by:

$$K_{obs} = \frac{K_{eq}}{(1 + (\beta/\alpha))} \qquad [6.3]$$

It can be seen from Equation 6.3 that the magnitude of K_{obs} will be less than K_{eq} for the process that promotes isomerization (i.e., $\beta/\alpha > 1$). Under these circumstances, the locations of the curves determining the response from the initial drug-receptor interaction are shifted to the left of the occupancy curve by a factor proportional to the magnitude of β/α (Fig 6-2).

The propensity of receptors to change from the R and R^* under the influence of an agonist is determined by the efficacy of the agonist. The production of R^* by an agonist can be considered a receptor-based signal for response, and it generally is termed *stimulus*, as defined by Stephenson (see Chapter 4). The magnitude of this property with the ability to promote

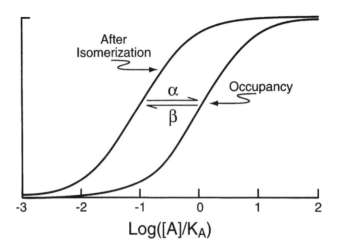

FIGURE 6-2. *The potentiation of agonist effect by receptor isomerization. The curve defining the stimulus produced by an agonist is shifted to the left of the receptor occupancy curve by the process of isomerization.*

receptor change (*intrinsic efficacy*) varies with different chemical structures; hence, it can be used as a molecular fingerprint for agonist-receptor pairs. The relative measurement of this property is an important aspect of receptor pharmacology, as the resulting constant transcends the system in which the receptor resides. This allows the study of agonists in surrogate systems and the prediction of activity in humans.

The stimulus produced by receptor activation by an agonist is processed by cellular machinery into a physiologic response. This machinery, where it pertains to the processing of a receptor-based signal, is referred to as the *stimulus-response mechanism(s)* of the cell. It translates the magnitude of the intrinsic efficacy message of the agonist into a signal that then is processed by the cellular cascades to observable response.

6.2.2 Heterotrimer Systems

Physiologic receptor systems primarily exist for control of cellular processes in response to exogenous stimuli. In a system in which the elements are ligand (drug *A*), receptor, and coupling mechanism, there are essentially four elements to be controlled: the concentration of ligand, the cell density of receptor, the magnitude of the equilibrium dissociation constant of the ligand-receptor complex, and the efficiency of translation of the receptor signal into response. The addition of an intermediary (i.e., receptor-coupling protein) increases the elements for possible cellular control. In these types of systems, there are two additional cellular control points—namely, the cellular quantity of the coupler and the equilibrium dissociation of the complex between activated receptor and coupler. A feature of such control mechanisms is promiscuity in that activated receptors are known to be able to interact with a number of couplers. Thus, the cell can control the type of response produced by receptors by the nature of the spectrum of couplers present. With such systems, cells can achieve tremendous diversity in the signals from a limited number of chemicals. Figure 6-3 depicts a common motif in receptor systems, the formation of hetero-trimers. The ligand-receptor complex (or activated receptor resulting from interaction with the ligand) interacts with another cellular component to form a heterotrimeric species of ligand-receptor-coupler, which then goes on to initiate response. Figure 6-4 illustrates signaling diversity in heterotrimeric systems. Whereas one single hormone can mediate two types of signals with two receptors that directly mediate a cellular response, those same two recep-tors may mediate a great many more responses with the intervention of a coupling protein and mixtures of effectors.

Great amplification can be achieved in such systems as well, as it often is not necessary for the trimeric species to be the responder (i.e., an activated

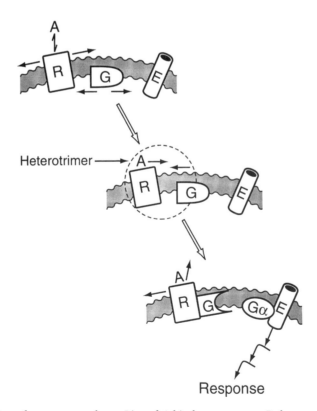

FIGURE 6-3. *The production of ternary complexes. Ligand A binds to a receptor R thus predisposing the AR complex to bind to another protein G. The ternary ARG complex dissociates to release part of the G-protein, which then goes on to activate the effector (E) and produce cellular response.*

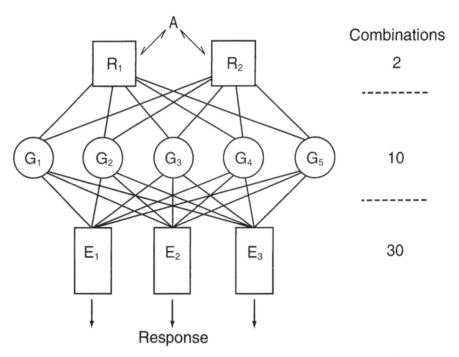

FIGURE 6-4. *Signaling diversity by mixing and matching of receptors (R), G-proteins, and effectors (E). A single ligand can initiate 2 separate responses when acting on 2 receptors, 10 different signals when the receptors interact with 5 different G-proteins, and 30 different signals when those G-proteins can interact with 3 different effectors.*

receptor may activate the coupler and then dissociate). This enables systems in which one activated receptor can activate numerous couplers. It also allows different temporal association between the initial receptor event and response in that the kinetics of decay of the coupler activation may be different from the kinetics of dissociation of the ligand-receptor complex. For example, the activation of sarcoplasmic reticular adenosine triphosphatase (ATPase) by adenosine 3':5'-cyclic phosphate (cyclic AMP) in cardiac cells stretches far beyond the cell surface receptor event that first initiates the process.

The effect of a second mass action coupling step after the initial interaction of a ligand and a receptor can result in tremendous signal amplification. Assuming that mass action kinetics apply, the production of the heterotrimeric species (denoted $[A \cdot R \cdot G]$, where the ligand is A, the receptor is R and the coupler is G) from a given concentration of ligand-receptor complex (denoted $[A \cdot R]$) is given by the following equation:

$$[A \cdot R \cdot G] = \frac{[A][R][G]}{[A]([G] + K_{AR}) + K_{AR}K_A} \qquad [6.4]$$

A feature of this equation is that K_{AR} (the equilibrium dissociation constant of the heterotrimer $[A \cdot R \cdot G]$) builds reserve into the system: That is, the maximal amount of $[A \cdot R \cdot G]$ complex for a given amount of $[R]$ and $[G]$ can be formed from a concentration of $[A]$ that is considerably less than the number of receptor sites. Thus, very low receptor occupancies can lead to maximal responses. This is an advantage in physiologic systems where the amount of circulating endogenous agonist (i.e., hormone or neurotransmitter) may be very low.

6.3 STIMULUS-RESPONSE MECHANISMS

The observed effect of a drug is the result of a complex interplay of mechanisms. The process begins with the drug binding to the receptor that produces an initial stimulus, which feeds into a cellular cascade. For example, the activation of a β-adrenergic receptor on the cell membrane will cause activation of membrane adenylate cyclase, which, in turn, will produce cytosolic cyclic AMP. This second messenger can go on to activate a number of biochemical processes within the cell, many of them interdependent on one another. For example, the cyclic AMP may go on to activate protein kinase, which can, in turn, activate phosphorylase kinase, to initiate a cascade of activation for phosphorylase b, glycogen, a number of substrates, and, finally, the production of glucose into the blood (Fig 6-5). Each of these biochemical processes has a threshold for activation and a maximal asymptote for steady-state response, (i.e., a dose-response curve). The nonlinearity of these sequential dose-response curves leads to a progressive potentiation of the signal. In this way, activation of an exceedingly small fraction of the receptor population can result in a strong physiologic signal from a receptor system. Under these circumstances, multiple receptor populations can be studied by dissection of the concentration ranges of selective drugs: That is, a very small but efficiently coupled population of receptors may be selectively activated by an agonist in the presence of a larger number of less efficiently coupled receptors. This concept can be useful in separating certain receptor populations from others (*vide infra*).

Commonly in biologic systems, the relationship between the input to the system and the output is hyperbolic in shape. The product of a succession of hyperbolae can be represented as a single hyperbolic function; thus, the entire stimulus-response cascade can be modeled with a single equation. A useful mathematic model of these processes is Equation 6.5:

$$Respsonse = \frac{Stimulus}{Stimulus + \beta} \qquad [6.5]$$

where β is a fitting parameter representing the amount of stimulus producing half the maximal response (in essence, the ED_{50}). The factor β becomes the

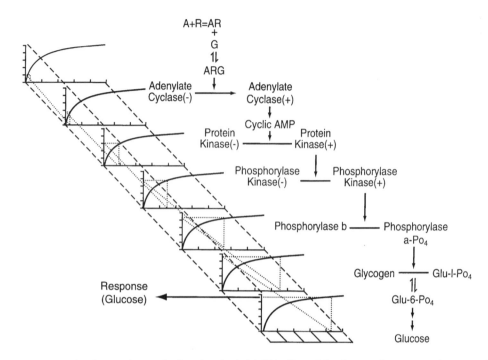

FIGURE 6-5. *A biochemical cascade showing the initial binding of the drug to the receptor (top reaction) through to the production of a biochemical cellular product (in this case, glucose; bottom reaction). Each step can be modeled by a hyperbolic function, and the product of each feeds into the next as the substrate. The dotted line shows how an initially very small receptor occupancy can result in nearly maximal response due to the high amplification of the system.*

location parameter for the dose-response curve driven by stimulus. Equation 6.5 is a mathematic representation of the stimulus-response mechanism for that particular tissue, whereby the magnitude of β represents the efficiency of transduction of receptor stimulus into tissue response. Thus, a highly efficient tissue that can produce a large response from a small stimulus would have a characteristically small value for β, whereas a less efficient tissue would have a larger value for β.

It can be shown mathematically that the location parameter [i.e., the abscissal value for half-maximal effect, such as the 50% effective concentration (EC_{50}) of a dose-response curve] for the result of two hyperbolic processes will lie to the left along the concentration axis of the K_A of the reaction that precedes it (Fig 6-6). Under these conditions:

$$EC_{50} = \frac{K_A}{((1+\beta)/\beta)} \qquad [6.6]$$

where β and K_A refer to the half-maximal concentrations for each of the singular functions. Because the denominator of Equation 6.6 is greater than

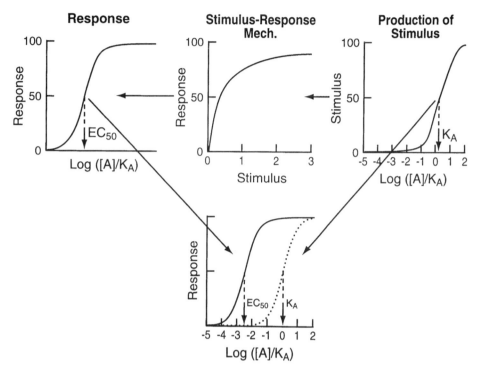

FIGURE 6-6. *The relationship between receptor stimulus and tissue response. A given concentration of agonist produces a stimulus; the location parameter for the curve describing this process is denoted as K_A (top right curve). This stimulus feeds into a hyperbolic function relating stimulus and response. Because of the skewed nature of this function (i.e., low x values yield high values of y), the response curve lies to the left of the stimulus curve; the location parameter for this curve is denoted EC_{50} (top left curve). The relationship between the stimulus curve and the response curve is shown in the lower center graph. The hyperbolic stimulus-response relationship potentiates the effects of the agonist.*

unity, then in all cases EC_{50} is less than K_A. This results in the condition whereby the dose-response curve for the complete process always will lie to the left of the dose-response curve for the preceding process. This is a general idea in pharmacology—namely, that the further away (in terms of the biochemical cascade connecting drug binding and tissue response) from the initial stimulus one views the result, the more sensitive will be the reading. If a third process were to be added to this scheme (with a location parameter ϕ; Fig 6-7), then it could be shown that the curve for the three-reaction process will lie to the left of the two-reaction process. This can be expressed mathematically by the fact that the E for the three-process scheme is calculated thus:

$$EC_{50} = \frac{K_A}{((1 + \phi\beta + \phi)/\phi\beta)} \qquad [6.7]$$

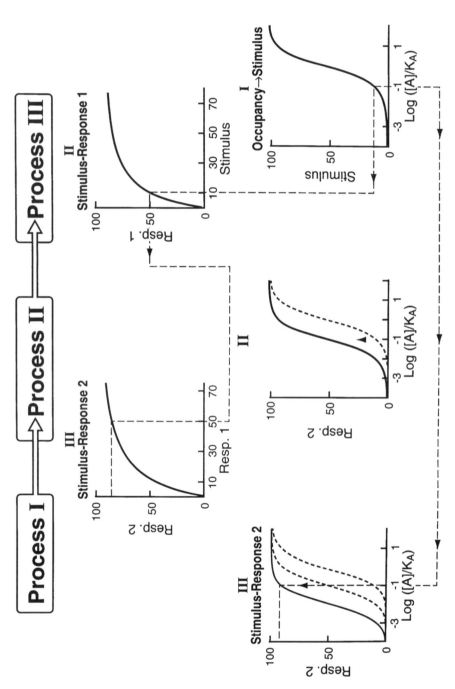

FIGURE 6-7. *The cascading effects of multiple hyperbolic processes. The addition of more hyperbolic functions between drug-receptor interaction curves and response curves produces further amplification. Note how the stimulus-response function I produces a shift to the left of the agonist curve (compare dotted and solid lines in graph II) whereas the addition of stimulus-response process II produces a further shift to the left of the agonist curve (graph III).*

A comparison of Equations 6.6 and 6.7 reveals that the denominator of the three-reaction sequence is larger than that for the two-reaction sequence by a factor of $(1/\phi\beta)$. Under these circumstances, the EC_{50} for the complete sequence will be less than the EC_{50} for any partial sequence.

It can be shown mathematically that the sensitivity of the total response of two or more hyperbolic processes will be greater than the sensitivity of any one of them. This idea is illustrated in Figure 6-8A in which a succession of biochemical reactions, emanating from the initial binding of the drug to the receptor, occurs in a cell. The initial binding curve is shown as well as hypothetical responses at various stages along the biochemical cascade. This process can lead to powerful amplification. For example, one β-adrenergic receptor in human neutrophils can generate 10,000 molecules of the second messenger cyclic AMP on activation. As seen in Figure 6-8B, the dose-response curve for the activation process viewed from vantage point 6 is shifted considerably to the left of the receptor occupancy curve. What this means in specific terms is that very small receptor occupancies are required to produce large responses at this point.

Figure 6-9 shows the relative proportion of receptors that must be activated by the agonist to produce a 50% response for the various processes. For the process shown in Figure 6-7B, the relative location of the occupancy and dose-response curves indicates that 0.0001% of the receptor population must be activated to induce a 50% response. Clearly, as the process is viewed nearer to the receptor occupation step, the larger the required activation is for receptor occupancy. Therefore, one advantage inherent in choosing highly amplified readouts for receptors is that the probability of selective effects of agonists is high because very low concentrations leading to very low receptor occupancies are required. This idea is used in Chapter 7 to choose the appropriate level of response for analysis of drug-receptor interaction.

Another advantage of using amplification cascades is that the responses to very weak agonists may be observed. As seen in Figure 6-8, usually the dose-response curves to an agonist are amplified the farther away from the receptor binding step the process is viewed. This can be exacerbated for very weak agonists to the point where the first steps in the cascade may produce stimuli that are unmeasurable, which is to say that they are so weak that they cannot be detected biochemically but nevertheless are of adequate strength to produce physiologic response after the biologic amplification. This poses a practical problem for the screening of new drug entities because usually the receptor screens are as simple as possible (i.e., a receptor responding to the initial stimulus mechanism). This is preferable because such systems are readily isolated and controlled (i.e., membrane fragments containing a receptor, G-protein, and adenylate cyclase for the production of cyclic AMP from ATP). However, a sizable signal is required, and therefore usually only fairly

Amplification of Weak Stimulis

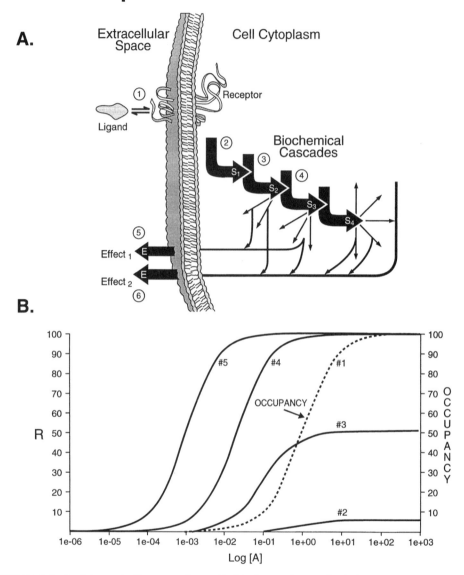

FIGURE 6-8. A. *Schematic diagram of cytosolic biochemical cascades linking drug-receptor interaction at the membrane to cellular response. Usually, an amplification of signal results from each biochemical step. B. The dose-response curves for the various steps are shown below the schematic diagram. There are advantages to viewing response production at many points along the stimulus-response chain.*

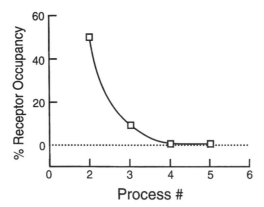

FIGURE 6-9. *The relative receptor occupancy required to produce 50% activation of sequential hyperbolic functions. After the first process (assume 50% activation requires 50% receptor occupancy), subsequent steps require activation of fewer and fewer receptors (i.e., by the fourth stimulus-response step, only 1% receptor occupancy at the membrane produces 50% activation of the process).*

powerful agonists will be detected. In the drug discovery process in which sampling from chemical space is tested randomly, it is likely that the initial drug lead will have only a hint of the desired efficacious property (i.e., that it will be very weak). Therefore, a highly amplified system would be a better choice for the detection of such activity. However, the counterargument to this is the fact that highly amplified biologic systems usually are complex (structured tissues, whole cells), which makes the control of variables more difficult.

Though in general the sensitivity of the system increases the further away from the initial receptor event the reaction is viewed, it is true also that complicating secondary biochemical reactions can be recruited into the cascade that may obfuscate the drug effect. Therefore, in practice, a balance between maximum sensitivity and minimal multiplicity in signal response is optimum for the study of drug-receptor effects.

6.4 THE ESTIMATION OF AGONIST EFFICACY

The magnitude of the sinistral translocation of the response curve (as determined by β/α) depends on the magnitude of the intrinsic efficacy of the agonist *and* the efficiency of translation of stimulus by the stimulus-response mechanism. Some tissues are extremely efficient (i.e., produce a large response for a comparably small stimulus) and some are not. For this reason, the absolute magnitude of the translocation cannot be used as a characteristic drug parameter, as this measurement would depend on the tissue in which the measurement was made. However, a relative measurement can be made between two agonists in the same tissue as the tissue-specific amplification characteristics would be common to both receptor stimuli. Under these circumstances, the only difference would be the magnitude of the intrinsic efficacy of the two agonists (see section 2.3, Null Methods, Chapter 2). This can be used as an operational measure of agonist intrinsic efficacy but only after the effect of affinity is neutralized.

The location of the dose-response curve along the concentration axis depends on four factors, two specific to the agonist and receptor pair and two for the receptor host system. The agonist-receptor specific factors are: affinity of the agonist for the receptor (K_A) and the intrinsic efficacy of the agonist for the receptor (β/α). The system-specific factors are: receptor density and the efficiency of translation of stimulus to response.

Measurement of the location of the dose-response curves for two agonists in the same tissues negates system-dependent effects. What remains to be accounted for are the relative affinities of the two agonists. This problem was overcome by the pharmacologist Robert Furchgott, who devised a method to measure operationally the relative efficacy of agonists (1). In this method, the response to the agonist is expressed as a function of the receptor occupancy, and the relative position of the "occupancy-response" curves becomes a measure of the relative power of the two agonists to produce response. Figure 6-10 shows how this technique negates the effects of receptor density, stimulus-response coupling, and affinity, and allows the comparison of the relative efficacy of two agonists.

6.4.1 Agonist Potency Ratios

The previous discussion illustrates how system factors can be canceled with null methods to express agonist activity in terms of the molecular parameters of affinity and efficacy. Furchgott showed how expression of response in terms of affinity allows for an operational measurement of relative efficacy (1). However, to accomplish this, an accurate measurement of the affinity constant of the agonist for the receptor must be known. Though techniques are available for measuring this constant, often it is not available. Under the latter circumstance, the location of an agonist dose-response curve still can function as a valuable measure for drug and receptor classification because under null conditions, they are the result of a combination of affinity and efficacy. Because these are unique molecular constants for the particular agonist and the particular receptor, agonist potency ratios can be, and have been, used as characteristic markers for agonists and receptors.

6.4.2 Efficacy-versus Affinity-Driven Agonists

As seen from the preceding discussion, both the affinity and efficacy of an agonist determine the location parameter of the dose-response curve to that

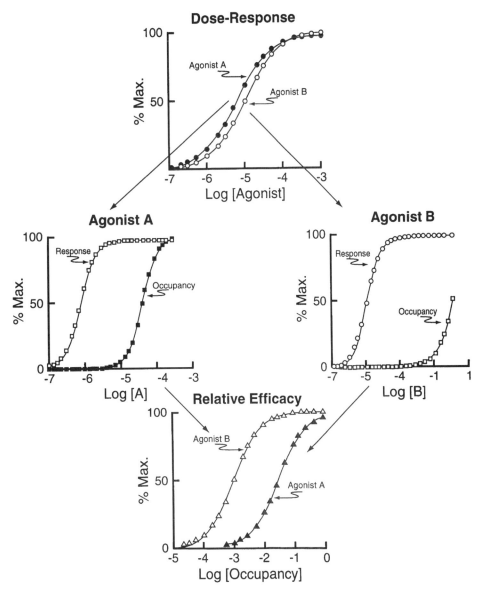

FIGURE 6-10. *Estimation of operational efficacy by the method of Furchgott. The top graph shows the relative potency of two agonists, A and B. The relationship of the dose-response curve of each agonist to its respective receptor occupancy curve is shown the next level down. As can be seen from this step, the response curve for agonist B is further to the left of its respective occupancy curve than is true for agonist A. Thus, showing that agonist B has a higher efficacy (i.e., a lower receptor occupancy results in a higher response). Expression of the response to each agonist as a function of the receptor occupancy is shown in the lowest curve. Now differences in affinity for the two agonists are accounted for, and the relative location of these curves reflects the relative efficacy of the two agonists. Note how the relative potency is different and reversed; that is, even though agonist A was more potent than agonist B in terms of concentration-response curves (top curve), agonist B is more efficacious than agonist A (bottom curve).*

agonist along the concentration axis. However, there is considerable difference between agonists whose potency is controlled primarily by affinity and those that are primarily driven by efficacy (2). Before this can be discussed, one must consider the spectrum of where along the concentration axis a dose-response curve to an agonist lies. Whereas stimulus-response mechanisms can potentiate weak signals and responses such that dose-response curves can be considerably shifted to the left of the curve defining receptor occupancy, diminution of signal capability cannot shift a dose-response curve to the right beyond the curve defining receptor occupancy. This is because, as the concentration of agonist enters this region, receptor occupancy becomes saturated and no further response can be generated from a system that has 100% receptor occupancy by an agonist. Figure 6-11 shows dose-response curves to an agonist in a system in which the response capability is progressively diminished. The dose-response curves collapse around the receptor occupancy curve for the agonist.

This has practical ramifications for agonists in different receptor systems. Figure 6-12 shows the dose-response curves to two theoretic agonists. Agonist I has a higher affinity for the receptor than agonist II but agonist II has a higher efficacy (i.e., produces more stimulus for a given receptor occupancy;

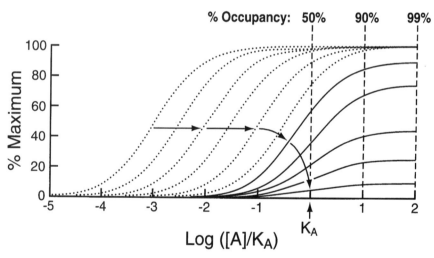

FIGURE 6-11. *The effects of progressive diminution of tissue response capability on the dose-response curve to an agonist. Decreasing responsiveness of the tissue system leads to parallel shifts to the right of the agonist dose-response curve. However, once the concentrations of agonist approach those required for maximal receptor occupancy, the curves do not shift to the right beyond that point but rather simply diminish in maximal asymptote. Dotted lines show the concentrations of agonist required for 50%, 90%, and 99% receptor occupancy. The dose-response curve to the agonist collapses around the region for maximal receptor occupancy.*

see Fig 6-12A,B). The overall location of the dose-response curves for the two agonists (after stimulus-response amplification by the tissue) is shown in Figure 6-12C. As these two agonists are tested in biologic systems of lower receptor-coupling efficiency, the response curve collapses toward the occupancy curve (as shown in Fig 6-11). However, because agonist II is of higher efficacy (such that the response curve is shifted further to the left of the occupancy curve), then reduction in stimulus translation will have a greater effect on the response to the lower-efficacy agonist I. The disparate effect on stimulus-response diminution for the two agonists is shown in Figure 6-12D and E. The relative responses to the two agonists in this less efficiently coupled tissue are shown in Figure 6-12F. Interestingly, whereas agonist I was more potent in the efficiently coupled tissue (Fig 6-12C), it is less effective in the less efficiently coupled tissue (Fig 6-12F). Further diminution of receptor coupling efficiency eliminates the response to agonist I (Fig 6-12G) and spares the response to the efficacy dominant Agonist II (Fig 6-12H). The relative effects in a poorly receptor-coupled tissue for the two agonists is shown in Figure 6-12I. This illustrates the relative robustness of responses to an efficacy-dominant agonist as opposed to a low-efficacy agonist that achieves potency by virtue of high affinity. In general, *efficacy-driven agonists are much more resistant to differences in stimulus-response coupling than are affinity-driven agonists.* Weak agonists that are potent by virtue of high affinity may show a greater vulnerability to loss of tissue viability.

6.5 THE MOLECULAR NATURE OF EFFICACY

Some drugs possess a unique chemical property known as *intrinsic efficacy,* that is inherent to their structure and it is through this property that such drugs transmit a biologic signal through the receptor to change the state of the cellular host. The molecular mechanisms through which this can occur are divided into two general categories: conformational selection and conformational induction (3). Conformational selection relates to a situation whereby an *active state of the receptor* (i.e., the state that, on its own, will trigger cellular signaling) *already exists in a library of receptor conformations* (albeit in very small quantities in the absence of agonist). The agonist then enters the reaction and shifts the population of receptors into a predominant active form by selective affinity to the active form. One way to view this is to think of proteins existing in two conformations (Fig 6-13). The "inactive" state of the receptor resides at a lower free energy than the active one; therefore, most of the receptors will gravitate to the inactive state. However, if an agonist selectively binds the active state of the receptor, then it effectively is removed from the equilibrium between the active and inactive receptor states and the population of receptors will again have to redistribute according to

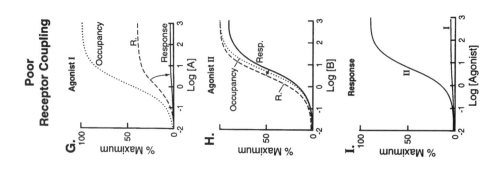

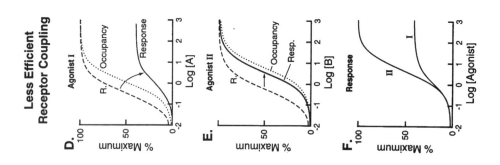

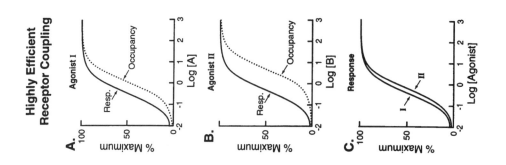

132

the natural energy levels. Therefore, more of the inactive receptor will migrate to the active state, according to the equilibrium dissociation constant. The net effect of this selective binding up of the active state is an increase in the number of receptors in the active state, either free or bound to agonist. The increase in the number of receptors in the active state will produce a physiologic response (see Fig 6-13).

This idea has been developed to describe the action of drugs on ion channels, which can exist in open and shut conformations. This allowed for the detection of the two states (i.e., one state each allowed ions to flow in or out of the cell, thus inducing a measurable current). It is worth discussing these ideas (two-state theory) in the context of agonism.

6.5.1 Two-State Theory

This model of drug receptors consists of the two receptor forms R_i and R_a, the latter being the "active" form of the receptor, which mediates physiologic response. The two forms are in equilibrium, defined by an activation constant K_{act} defined as $[R_i]/[R_a]$. A ligand has affinity for each. The equilibrium dissociation constant of the ligand and inactive form is denoted K, and of the active form K/α. The behavior of this system is described by the following equation:

$$\rho_{R_a} = \frac{1}{1 + K_{act}(1 + [A]/K)/(1 + \alpha[A]/K)} \qquad [6.8]$$

where ρ_{Ra} is the fraction of receptors in the R_a form. It can be seen from this equation that if a ligand has a higher affinity for R_a (i.e., if $\alpha > 1$), then as the concentration of A increases, so too does the proportion of receptors in the R_a form ($\rho_{Ra} \rightarrow 1$). Before consideration of the effects of a drug on this system,

---

FIGURE 6-12. *The effects of diminishing tissue response capability on the effects of efficacy-driven versus affinity-driven agonists. In a system of highly efficient stimulus-response coupling, both agonists produce maximal response. Two agonists are shown: agonist I has high affinity but low efficacy (A) and agonist II has a high efficacy but low affinity (B). In the highly coupled system, agonist I is slightly more potent (C). In the middle panel, the effects of both agonists in a less highly efficient receptor-coupling system are shown. The affinity-driven agonist (agonist I) produces only partial agonism as it has low efficacy (D). The efficacy-driven agonist still produces maximal response (E). The lower middle panel shows that agonist I produces partial agonism (but is still more potent than agonist II; F). The set of graphs furthest to the right show the effects of the agonists in a poorly coupled tissue. Under these circumstances, agonist I has insufficient efficacy to produce any response (G) whereas the agonist of higher efficacy (agonist II) can still produce response (H). It can be seen from this simulation that the efficiency of receptor coupling can produce a system in which the relative potencies of two agonists can reverse completely (I).*

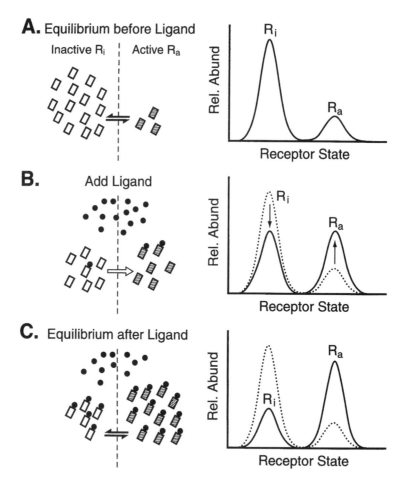

FIGURE 6-13. *Changes in receptor states due to selective agonist affinity. A. The system is such that most of the receptors are in the inactive (R_i) state. The relative proportions of the receptors in each state are shown by two histograms on the right. B. A ligand is added that has a higher affinity for the active (R_a) state than the inactive (R_i) state. By virtue of this selective affinity, the equilibrium of the system begins to shift toward the production of more active state receptor (R_a). C. At equilibrium, more of the receptors are trapped in the active state because of the selective binding action of the agonist.*

the different states of the system itself should be explored. Therefore, when the drug concentration is zero, Equation 6.8 reduces to the following expression:

$$\rho_{R_a} = \frac{1}{1 + K_{act}} \qquad [6.9]$$

From this equation it can be seen that if the natural state of the receptors is in the active form (i.e. $[R_a] \gg [R_i]$), then ρ_{Ra} will tend toward unity. Thus, the magnitude of K_{act} will determine the set point of the system, which a drug will change by its presence.

There can be three kinds of drug activities imposed on this system: 1) those with preferential affinity for R_a that therefore increase R_a ($\alpha > 1$); 2) those with equal affinity for R_i and R_a ($\alpha = 1$); and 3) those with preferential affinity for R_i over R_a ($\alpha < 1$). Clearly, if α equals 1, then the presence of the drug will not change $[R_a]/[R_i]$ (ρ_{Ra}). In contrast, the dependence of ρ_{Ra} on the concentration of a drug with α equal to 10 is shown in Figure 6-14A. The effects of A for three different set points for the system ($K_{act} = 100, 1, 0.001$) are shown to illustrate the overriding effects of the system on drug response. It can be seen from this figure that if the system already has most of the receptors in the R_a form, then very little effect of a drug with α in excess of 1 will be observed. At other set points where the basal amounts of R_a are less than complete, the drug increases this to $[R_a]/[R_i]$ toward unity.

A contrasting activity is seen with drugs that destabilize the R_a form (i.e., where $\alpha < 1$). Here the ligand prefers the R_i form of the receptor and shifts the equilibrium toward it. Figure 6-14B shows a mirror image of the activity shown in Figure 6-14A in that, when the proportion of R_a is high ($K_{act} = 0.001$), a drug for which α is less than 1 will depress the fraction ρ_{Ra} toward zero. Similarly, a mirror-image dose-response curve is observed for systems in which half of the receptors are in the R_a form. Only in systems in which none of the receptors are in the R_a form will a drug with α of less than 1 have no direct effects.

It can be seen from these examples that the interplay between the intrinsic molecular activity of the drug (i.e., the differential affinity for the two protein conformations denoted by α) and the set point of the system is paramount. A given drug might have a pronounced activity or no activity in two different systems, depending on the magnitudes of α and K_{act}. Figure 6-15A shows a surface for a drug with a differential affinity favoring the R_a form ($\alpha > 1$) in systems of varying values for K_{act}. It can be seen from this figure that there are regions of system override and system sensitivity. Figure 6-15B shows the same type of surface for a drug that destabilizes the R_a form ($\alpha < 1$). Basically, the same ideas apply except that the effects are mirror images of those seen with drugs for which α is greater than 1.

An important aspect of two-state theory is the effect of α on the maximal response of a given drug. Though it might be supposed that a drug that preferentially binds to the R_a form of the receptor eventually will convert all the receptors into that form, this may not be the case if the drug has a substantial affinity for the R_i form as well. Under these circumstances, the drug also will freeze some of the receptors into the R_i form, and a set ratio of the two will emerge at saturating concentrations of drug. The maximal response to a drug can be calculated using Equation 6.8 at $[A] \to \infty$. Under these circumstances, equation 6.8 reduces to the following:

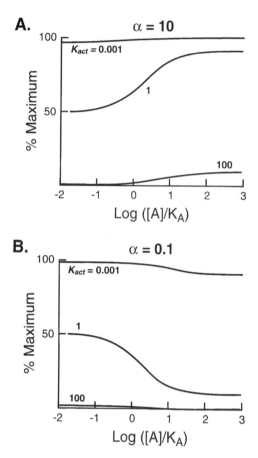

FIGURE 6-14. *The effects of ligands on two-state systems. A. The effects of a positive agonist ($\alpha > 1$, where the agonist has a higher affinity for the active state of the receptor). In quiescent systems ($K_{act} = 100$, most of the receptors in the inactive state), the ligand produces a small increase in the active state. B. In a system, in which an equal proportion of receptors are in the inactive and active states ($K_{act} = 1$), the ligand is able to produce a total change to the active state. In highly spontaneously active systems ($K_{act} = 0.001$), little effect with this ligand is seen because most of the receptors are already in the active state. C. The same analysis shown in A with an inverse agonist (i.e., ligand that prefers the inactive state) ($\alpha = 0.1$). In a system where most of the receptors are in the active state ($K_{act} = 0.001$), a small decrease in response is observed with the ligand. In a system with equal proportions of active and inactive receptor ($K_{act} = 1$), a prominent inverse agonism is seen. In a quiescent system ($K_{act} = 100$), no effect is seen because most of the receptors are already in the inactive state.*

$$\rho_{R_a} = \frac{1}{1 + K_{act}/\alpha} \qquad [6.10]$$

Here again the interplay between the system and the drug can be seen. In systems where a great many of the receptors are in the R_i form, even a drug with a very selective affinity for the R_a state ($\alpha \gg 1$) may still not increase ρ_{Ra}.

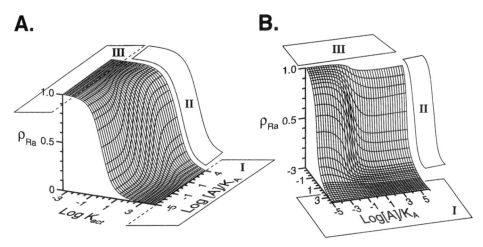

FIGURE 6-15. *The interrelationships between system set points and two-state ligands.* A. *Effects of a positive agonist (α > 1) on various systems (variable values of K_{act}). In region III, the system already is at maximally activated receptor; thus no further effect of the agonist is seen (low values of K_{act}). In region II, the system allows the ligand to modify the relative proportions of receptors. In region I, the system is shut down to the point whereby the agonist cannot increase the proportion of receptors in the active state.* B. *The effects of an inverse agonist (α < 1). In region III, a large proportion of the receptors are in the active state, but the ligand still can produce a small reduction. In region II, the system is more responsive (moderate values of K_{act}). In region I, the system is in the inactive state and cannot be further depressed.*

Thus, a system that is in a very inert state $[R_i] >> [R_a]$ may still not respond well even to a powerful agonist. As can be seen from Equation 6.10, a wide variety of combinations of K_{act} and α will result in ratios of active and inactive receptor of less than unity.

6.5.2 Conformational Induction

The other mechanism for agonism, *conformational induction,* is more difficult to describe in thermodynamic terms as it implies that the *active state of the receptor is not present until the agonist is present.* Thus, the agonist, by the act of binding, deforms the receptor into another conformational state, which goes on to produce response. There is less direct evidence for this mechanism, although there are data to suggest that some receptor states do not exist until a drug is bound to them. Instead of selective affinity for the active state, the agonist would be thought of as having an electronic configuration that brings it near to one other binding elements in the receptor that normally would not be associated, (or otherwise translocated), to induce a conformational change that then activates receptor-coupling elements to produce cellular response. The change produced by an agonist can be thought of as an isomerization of the receptor, and this idea can be used to describe the behavior of agonists in receptor systems.

6.5.3 Receptor Protein Energy Landscapes

The concepts of conformational selection and induction merge somewhat in the idea that receptors, like all proteins, probably exist in a large number of tertiary conformations (not only in an active and inactive state). Under these circumstances, thermal energy causes the receptor to continually adopt various conformations. This can be conceptualized as the receptor moving along a surface of energy wells, each well being a definitive conformation; such surfaces are referred to as *energy landscapes* (Fig 6-16A). At any one instant, the population of receptors can be defined as various fractions frozen in the various conformations (Fig 6-16B). Agonists may induce an enrichment of the various conformational states by selective affinity (conformational selection). It is not clear whether all agonists produce the same steady-state milieu of receptor conformations (Fig 6-16C, D). This opens the possibility that drug effect can be agonist-selective even when the agonists involved act on the same receptor. The therapeutic potential for this effect is great because it allows for organ-selective receptor effects.

6.5.4 Conformational Selection and Induction on Energy Landscapes

The idea that agonists could either choose active receptor conformations (conformational selection) or create them (conformational induction) was introduced first into receptor theory as a set of opposing views of agonism. However, examination of the energy landscape concept shows that they are compatible with each other and are, in fact, extremes of the same molecular mechanism. Thus, the selection and stabilization of a receptor conformation, rarely found in the absence of the agonist, would be indistinguishable from receptor induction as the conformation would be undetectable in the absence of agonist. Therefore, it would appear that the agonist "created" the conformation. This is preferable in terms of energy, because it would not require the receptor to form an energetically unfavorable conformation.

6.6 INDIRECT AGONISM

Drugs may also produce response by release of endogenous direct agonists (see Chapter 5) or modulation of ongoing physiologic processes. In these systems, an augmentation of a basal physiologic process (i.e., by making it more efficient) produces an apparently new response. One example of this is by ligand binding to a site on the receptor different from that used by the endogenous agonist (see Fig 1-5C). Such ligands are referred to as *allotopic effectors* (see Chapter 1). Activity from this mechanism is more difficult to

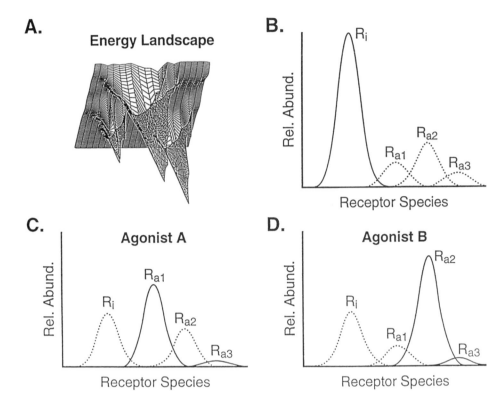

FIGURE 6-16. *Receptor active states as part of an energy landscape. A. Depiction of energy wells describing different conformational states of receptors. Thermal energy causes the receptor to traverse this landscape and fall into various energy wells according to various equilibrium constants. B. A snapshot depicting the relative proportion of receptors in various states. In this case, most of the receptors are in the inactive (R_i) state and have the capability of forming three active states. C. The addition of a saturating concentration of an agonist that selects a certain number of active states produces steady-state elevations of two of the active states at the expense of the inactive state. D. Another agonist may select another collection of active states, producing an enrichment of those other states.*

characterize and more variable across systems because the magnitude of the response to the allotopic effector is inexorably tied to the basal activity of the system. An example of an allotopic effector agonist is shown in Figure 6-17. As can be seen from this figure, the dose-response curve for the endogenous agonist producing the basal effect is shifted to the left by the allotopic effector. At any given level of endogenous basal tone, the allotopic effector produces an elevation of the existing tone, thereby eliciting a response. However, it can be seen also in this figure that this type of agonism has its limits in that if the system already is driven to maximal response by endogenous agonist, then an allotopic effector will have no further effect. If no basal tone is available to potentiate, then similarly, an allotopic effector agonist will have no effect.

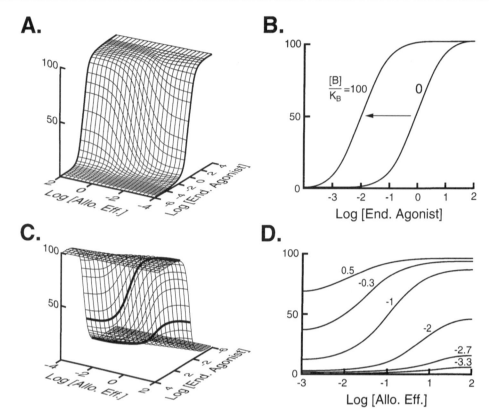

FIGURE 6-17. *Allosteric effectors as agonists. A. The array of different interactions between an allosteric effector A that increases the efficiency of activation of an endogenous agonist and the concentration of endogenous agonist present in the medium. B. The two darkened curves in A are shown. These represent the response to the endogenous agonist in the absence ([B]/K_B = 0) and presence ([B]/K_B = 100) of the allosteric effector agonist. The saturating concentration of allosteric effector B causes a 100-fold shift to the left of the curve to the endogenous agonist. C. Curves shown in A from the vantage point of the allosteric effector agonist. Two curves to the allosteric effector agonist are highlighted, one in the absence of a low concentration of endogenous agonist (response begins at 0 and increases to 40%) and the other in the presence of a concentration of endogenous agonist which itself produces a basal response of 30%. In this case, the allosteric effector agonist increases the response to the maximal asymptote. D. The effects of various levels of endogenous agonist (shown as log values from 0.5 to -3.0) on the observed response to the allosteric effector agonist.*

6.7 SYNOPSIS

The following ideas were presented in this chapter:

- Agonism is the production of a change of state of a biologic system by the action of an agonist on a receptor. Agonists can initiate, inhibit, modulate, or potentiate biologic processes to produce response.

- Direct agonists produce response by causing receptor isomerization (producing an activated receptor form). The process of receptor isomerization distorts the observed affinity of the agonist to one describing the complete reaction of binding plus isomerization.

- Agonists produce a receptor stimulus that then is processed by the stimulus-response mechanisms of biologic tissues. These processes are composed of sequential biochemical reactions that can be modeled by sequential hyperbolic functions.

- Great signaling diversity and amplification can be achieved by interacting components such as heterotrimers.

- As tissue response is viewed farther from the initial drug-receptor interaction, the signal usually is amplified, and the potency of the agonist producing the responses increases with each step.

- Extraordinary selectivity can be achieved by the study of tissue response, as low levels of receptor activation, by virtue of stimulus-re sponse amplification, can result in powerful signals.

- Agonist potency depends on system factors (receptor density and stimulus-response coupling) and drug factors (affinity and efficacy). Whereas agonist potency ratios cancel system effects and can be used for classification, the measurement of efficacy (i.e., by the Furchgott method) provides a better idea of agonist power.

- Efficacy-driven agonists are more resistant to system effects than are affinity-driven agonists.

- In molecular terms, agonists may induce receptor isomerization (agonism) through protein conformational induction or selection. For the latter mechanism, the system set point can override the effects of the agonist.

- Indirect agonists may release endogenous agonists to produce response.

REFERENCES

1. Besse JC, Furchgott RF. Dissociation constants and relative efficacies of agonists acting on alpha-adrenergic receptors in rabbit aorta. J Pharmacol Exp Ther 1972;197:68–78.
2. Kenakin TP. The relative contribution of affinity and efficacy to agonist activity: organ selectivity of noradrenaline and oxymetazoline with reference to the classification of drug receptors. Br J Pharmacol 1984;81:131–143.

3. Burgen ASV. Conformational changes and drug action. Fed Proc 1981;40:2723–2728.

FURTHER READING

Costa T, Ogino Y, Munson PJ, et al. Drug efficacy at guanine nucleotide-binding regulatory protein-linked receptors: thermodynamic interpretation of negative antagonism and of receptor activity in the absence of ligand. 1992;41:549–560.

Furchgott RF. The use of β-haloalkylamines in the differentiation of receptors and in the determination of dissociation constants of receptor agonist complexes. In: Harper NJ, Simmonds AB eds. Advances in drug research, vol 3. New York: Academic,1966:21–55.

Lefkowitz RJ, Cotecchia S, Samama P, Costa T. Constitutive activity of receptors coupled to guanine regulatory proteins. Trends Pharmacol Sci 1993;14:303–307.

Drug-Response Measurement Systems: Signal Strength, Stability, and Selectivity

THIS CHAPTER deals with the practicalities involved in the measurement of drug-receptor interaction. The most direct way of taking such measurements is by monitoring the amount of radiolabeled drug-receptor complex formed by mixing fixed quantities of radioactive drug and receptor (biochemcial binding, section 7.2). Also, data on the physiologic effects of drugs on biologic receptor systems can be obtained from a variety of functional assays (section 7.3). The prerequisites for the acquisition of reliable data is the measurement of strong, stable, and clean responses to drugs (sections 7.3.1 and 7.3.2). The various assays commonly used to measure functional response are given in section 7.3.3. Section 7.4 discusses metameters used in pharmacology to measure and compare biologic effects. Responses to drugs can be measured as they happen (real time) or after they occur by assay of the product of the drug-receptor interaction accumulated over a set time (stop-time). The advantages and disadvantages of each approach are given in section 7.5. These ideas are summarized at the end of the chapter (section 7.6).

7.1 MEASUREMENT OF DRUG-RECEPTOR INTERACTION

It is axiomatic that relevant information about drugs and receptors will be obtained from monitoring the interactions between the two. In general, there are two broad experimental approaches used to do this—specifically, the measurement of the binding of drugs to receptor populations (biochemical binding studies) and the measurement of the cellular (or subcellular) responses produced by the interaction of drugs with receptors (functional studies). Biochemical binding studies are concerned with the behavior of complete populations of receptors, whereas functional studies can view partial populations (Fig 7-1). It is worth considering the relative advantages and disadvantages of both of these approaches.

Figure 7-2A shows a curve of a ligand binding to three populations of receptors. Receptor population 1 is most sensitive to the ligand, but there is less of this receptor than of the other two. Shown also in this figure are the individual binding curves to each of the three populations as well as the curve for total binding to all of the receptors. It can be seen from this figure

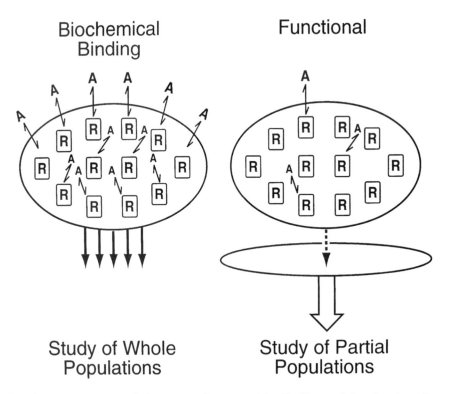

FIGURE 7-1. *The relative receptor populations generally accessed by binding and functional studies, respectively. Usually only a small proportion of the receptors need be activated to yield a measurable functional response.*

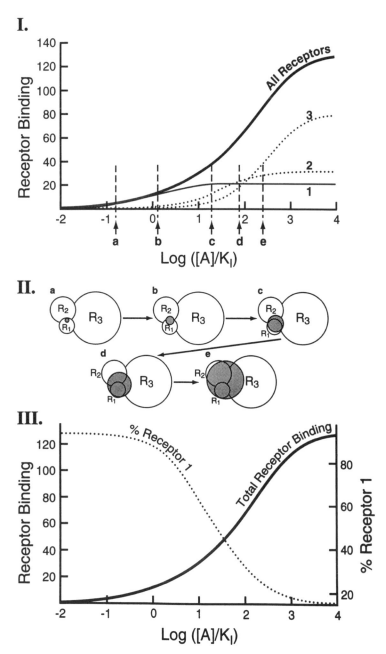

FIGURE 7-2. *The interaction of a ligand with three different receptor populations. A. The ligand binds to three populations with differential affinity. It is most potent for population 1, but this population contains fewer total receptors than the other two populations. B. Circles show the relative size of the three populations of receptor and the relative interaction of various concentrations of the ligand (in the darkened circle) with each population. Panel a shows a very low concentration of ligand; it almost exclusively interacts with population 1. As the concentration of ligand increases (panels b–e), the ligand interaction spills over into the other receptor populations. C. The total bound receptor is shown in the solid-line curve. The percentage of the binding to population 1 is shown in the dotted-line curve. As the concentration of ligand increases, the relative percent binding to only population 1 declines.*

that whereas low concentrations of ligand bind primarily to receptor population 1, higher concentrations spill over into the other receptor populations. Moreover, as this occurs, because the secondary receptor populations (populations 2 and 3) are larger than receptor 1, as more ligand is added, more binds to those receptors than to the primary population. The relative binding of given concentrations of ligand (denoted by the darkened circle) to the three receptor populations is shown in Figure 7-2B. Not only do higher concentrations of ligand bind to the secondary receptor populations, but also the center of the darkened circle shifts, indicating that the selectivity of the ligand for receptor 1 is lost at higher concentrations. Figure 7-2C shows the diminishing fraction of total receptor due to receptor population 1 with increasing concentration of ligand. In general, this illustrates the difficulty in retaining specificity of drug effect with binding studies. A ligand must be extraordinarily selective to achieve total binding to a receptor population without interacting with other sites. In this sense, the study of portions of receptor populations (as can be done with functional assays) has advantages. However, binding studies can furnish invaluable data about the stoichiometry of drug-receptor interactions and the nature of the species formed. Moreover, the drug-receptor complex can be studied directly, allowing the shapes of binding curves to be interpreted in molecular terms.

7.2 BIOCHEMICAL BINDING STUDIES

A great deal of information about drug-receptor interaction can be obtained from the study of the quantity of and the manner in which a radiolabeled drug binds to a receptor (1). In general, a given concentration of radiolabeled drug is equilibrated with a preparation containing receptors (i.e., whole cells, fragments of cell membrane) for a set time period (sufficient for the receptor and the drug to come to binding equilibrium with each other). Then, the receptor preparation is physically isolated and the radioactivity quantified. The magnitude of the radioactive signal is directly proportional to the amount of drug bound to the receptor and, because the concentration of drug is known, a dose-response curve for binding to the receptor can be obtained (Fig 7-3). Most radiolabeled drugs bind to other sites on the membrane in addition to receptors (termed *nonspecific binding*); therefore, parallel experiments are run in which a drug known to bind to the receptors is present in a concentration that will protect the receptor population from being labeled with the radiolabel. If the radioactivity from this nonspecific binding is subtracted from the total binding (receptors plus nonspecific sites), the yield is the radioactivity associated only with the receptor population.

The binding of a radioligand to a huge population of nonspecific binding (nsb) sites of mixed origin can be approximated by a linear relationship

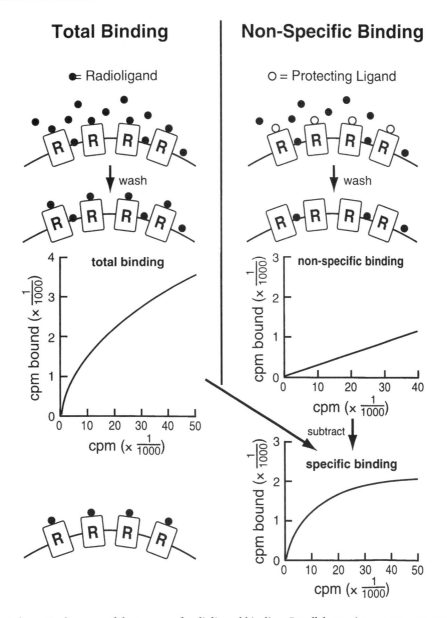

FIGURE 7-3. *Schematic diagram of the process of radioligand binding. Parallel experiments are run, one involving incubation of the receptor preparation with radioligand and one with radioligand in the presence of a saturating concentration of nonradioactive receptor active ligand that will serve to protect only the receptors from binding with the radioligand. The two curves represent the result of this process repeated with a range of concentrations of radioligand. Subtraction of the two curves yields the amount of radioligand bound only to the receptors (specific binding; bottom curve).*

between the concentration of radioligand and the amount of nonspecific binding:

$$nsb = k\,[A^*] \qquad\qquad [7.1]$$

The total binding of a radioligand to a defined population of receptors (where binding is saturable) and a much larger population of other nonreceptor sites (nonspecific binding) can be modeled by a summation of the Langmuir adsorption isotherm and a linear model of nonspecific binding:

$$\text{Total binding} = \frac{[A^*]B_{max}}{[A^*] + K_d} + k[A^*] \qquad\qquad [7.2]$$

An accurate way to accomplish this is to fit the curve for total binding and nonspecific binding (determined separately) simultaneously to Equations 7.2 and 7.3, respectively. Under these circumstances the maximal asymptote for receptor binding (B_{max}) and the sensitivity of the receptor preparation to the radioligand (K_d, the equilibrium dissociation constant of the radioligand receptor complex) can be estimated mathematically and compared to receptor models.

One practical consideration of binding studies is the requirement that the process of binding not alter the free concentration of ligand (see Chapter 5). To ensure this, the binding of a given concentration of ligand is measured at various amounts of receptor material (usually cell membrane containing the receptor). As the amount of receptor becomes large enough to deplete the amount of radioligand, the amount bound reaches a limit. This is denoted by a curvature of the concentration-binding curve for increasing amounts of receptor (Fig 7-4A). Noting that this is the region where binding alters the free radioligand concentration, experiments must be done in the linear region of this curve (Fig 7-4A).

Another consideration in binding studies is that the binding adhere to first order kinetics. Thus, the binding must reach a maximum with increasing time and be reversible on washing with drug-free medium (Fig 7-4B). Because binding experiments are done in stop-time (*vide infra*), the receptor preparation must be equilibrated with the ligands for a period of time adequate to reach equilibrium (Fig 7-4B).

The total amount of radioligand bound to the preparation that can be displaced by a specific protecting ligand for the receptor population defines the specific binding of the preparation (i.e., the relative quantity of the total binding that is due to receptors). For some adherent radioligands (or some specifically adherent receptor membrane preparations), the nonspecific binding may be very high thus defining a relatively minor amount of the signal to receptors (Fig 7-5A). Under these circumstances, the reliable definition of

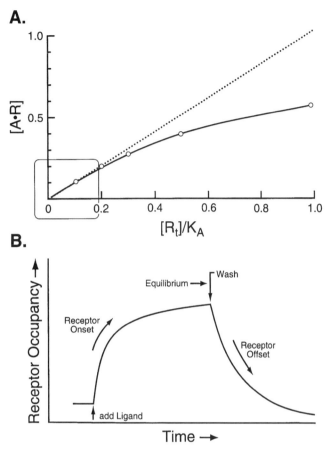

FIGURE 7-4. *Equilibrium conditions for binding studies. A. The effect of increasing receptor concentration on the production of a complex between the receptor and the radioligand. As the receptor concentration increases, the binding depletes the amount of free radioligand until saturation occurs (i.e. there is no further radioligand in the medium left to bind and no further ligand-receptor complex is formed). For accurate estimation of parameters and use of receptor models, the signal and receptor concentration needs to be kept in the linear portion of this curve (inside the square area). B. The kinetics of equilibration of a radioligand with receptor. Experiments must be done after a steady state has been attained (equilibrium plateau). Moreover, binding should be reversible in that washing with drug-free medium should remove the radioligand from the receptor.*

receptor-binding events is difficult and subject to statistical error. However, some ligands are extremely selective for receptors over nonspecific sites, and the nonspecific binding is extremely low. Under these circumstances, most of the signal is attributable to receptors (Fig 7-5B). In general, experimental conditions should be optimized for maximum specific binding.

As discussed previously, direct measurement of the amount of complex formed between a drug and its receptor allows the shapes of dose-response

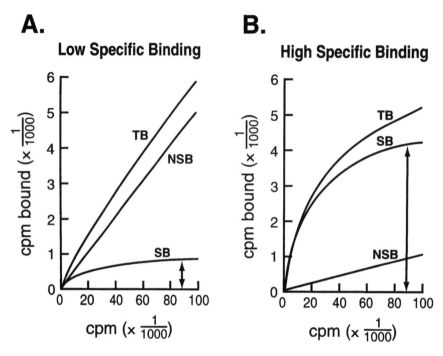

FIGURE 7-5. *Different levels of specific binding in radioligand-binding experiments. A. The total binding (TB) approaches the nonspecific binding (NSB). This preparation has a low level of specific binding (SB). B. The difference between total binding and nonspecific binding is large, indicating a large population of receptors and a high level of specific binding.*

curves to be interpreted in molecular terms. In general, these analyses all compare the observed binding to the Langmuir adsorption isotherm (see Chapter 3) model for a single ligand binding to a single population of identical sites. Deviation from this model can be interpreted in terms of multisite populations or multistate populations, whereby a receptor converts to another entity on binding. The discernment of deviations from the simple model can be greatly aided by statistics; this is discussed more fully in Chapter 9.

7.3 FUNCTIONAL STUDIES

7.3.1 Types of Drug Response

Living biologic systems usually have characteristic indicators of their physiologic state (e.g., basal rate of metabolism, hydrogen ion extrusion, tonic muscular tone). Biologic drug response can be measured once an appropriate physiologic indicator is identified. There are two basic requirements for this factor: 1) The signal-to-noise ratio must be adequate to differentiate drug-induced change, and 2) the basal activity must be stable to allow measurement of change.

The actual magnitude of a drug response, assuming that the sensitivity of the measuring tools is sufficient to detect the signal, is not nearly as important as its relationship to the random noise of the preparation. The first requirement encountered is the basal stability of the receptor system.

7.3.2 System Stability

In general, the measurement of biologic drug response requires a complex system of receptors for recognition of the drug and translation of information and a transduction system to amplify the stimulus and produce a measurable signal. Often, this latter process involves the augmentation of an ongoing basal process within the cell. For example, the second messenger, cyclic AMP, is present in the cytosol as a result of the basal functioning of adenylate cyclase. Similarly, seven-transmembrane receptors exist in partial populations that are spontaneously active and thus produce low levels of basal biologic activity. In general, biologic experiments have a characteristic window of stability and viability either side of which is unsuitable for reliable data. Often the preparation of the system in vitro (e.g., plating of cell culture, dissection of isolated tissues) is traumatic and the resulting basal activity of the system is unsuitably unstable and variable. Thus, to achieve stability, an equilibration period must be allowed before the experiment (Fig 7-6). Preparations vary in the length of time they remain stable, but inevitably the differences between

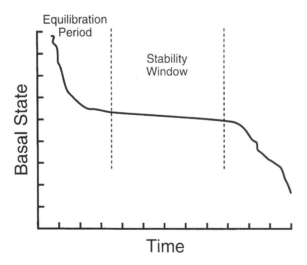

FIGURE 7-6. *Stability windows for biologic preparations. When biologic systems are prepared for in vitro study, a period of recovery from trauma is usually needed (equilibration period), followed by a stable period during which experimental data can be collected, followed by a period of declining viability.*

natural and in vitro conditions lead to a deterioration of function (see Fig 7-6). The rates for such deterioration also can be variable; therefore, data collected in this period are unreliable.

The tenet of independent experiments in different receptor preparations is that the sensitivity and responsiveness of the *biologic system has not changed throughout the course of the experiment*. It often is difficult to obtain data to support this assumption, so it must be accepted without qualification. There are two broad approaches used to reduce potential errors for system instability. The first is to "correct" for changes in basal function within the experiment. For example, if the resting state of the preparation can be deduced from the baseline response in the absence of drug, then a drift in the baseline can be extrapolated and assumed in the calculation of drug response. If the drift is linear it is more easily predicted than if it is the more commonly observed hyperbolic deterioration of baseline (Fig 7-7).

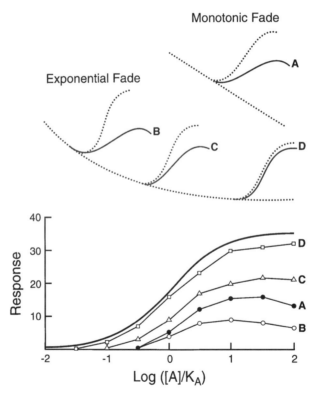

FIGURE 7-7. *The effects of moving baselines on dose-response curves. Baselines can decline monotonically (straight line, upper tracing) or exponentially (lower tracing). If a dose-response curve is obtained on these moving baselines, the curves denoted A to D would result. The bottom dose-response curves are the experimentally obtained curves compared to the true curve (i.e., no fading baseline). As can be seen from this figure, early exponential fade produces the most pronounced error. In general, fading baselines affect the maximal asymptote but not the location parameter of dose-response curves.*

A second type of correction is via a secondary "control" experimental preparation whereby no drug treatment is obtained and only the basal function is monitored. This may be more hazardous than an intraexperimental correction as the variability between two different preparations is incorporated as well. This can be serious because different preparations may deteriorate at very different rates. For example, it can be assumed that in a biologic system consisting of a collection of cells (i.e., cell culture), after a period of viability, some of the cells begin to die and the overall rate of cell death is exponential (i.e., $\rho = e^{-kt}$ where k is a rate constant for cell death and ρ is the fraction of cells remaining viable). Assuming differences in the dependence of total system responsiveness to drugs on viable cell number (i.e., one culture may be more efficiently coupled than another or may have a different number of expressed receptors), exceedingly small differences in k can lead to disparate changes in drug sensitivity in two independent preparations. The predicted effects of exponential cell death on dose-response curves is shown in Figure 7-8. Given the complex relationship between cell viability and agonist potency, it is unlikely that one system would be a good control for changes in basal responsiveness between tissues. In general, the most reliable data are obtained from systems of known stability, and all data should be collected well within stability windows.

All functional receptor preparations have a definite window of responsiveness—that is, a range of drug concentrations wherein the response primarily is due to the activation of a single receptor population and the resulting response is due only to activation of that population. When this concentration range is exceeded, secondary effects of drugs are observed. In many instances, these secondary effects can be visualized by a clear change in the slope or maximal asymptote of the dose-response curve (Fig 7-9). In other cases, a change in the shape of the curve may indicate secondary effects. Figure 7-10A shows a series of dose-response curves to an agonist that activates a secondary response mechanism at concentrations beyond 20 units. In this case, interventions selective for the receptor of interest that move the dose-response curve to these higher concentrations (such as receptor antagonism or loss of biologic sensitivity of the system to receptor stimulation) push the curve against an apparent wall beyond which the curve will not progress. The resulting effects on the observed curves show an increased slope and loss of the sigmoidal shape that was indicative of single receptor activation (Fig 7-10B).

7.3.3 Functional Drug-Receptor Assays

Pharmacology is rich with a heritage of the use of isolated tissues to measure drug effect. For the most part, the use of these systems was expedient in that these were the only assays available in early years to assess biologic response. However, as technology has allowed, the stimulus-response cascade has been dissected until, at present, there are numerous points along many cascades that

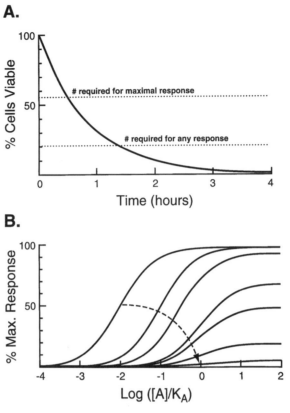

FIGURE 7-8. *Effects of exponential cell death on dose-response curves to agonists. A. Percent of viable cells with time of experiment in a biologic preparation. The top dotted line refers to the minimal number of cells required to generate the maximal response to the agonist. The bottom dotted line indicates the minimal number of cells required to produce any response to the agonist. B. Dose-response curves to the agonist with increasing time. In general, tissues lose sensitivity (as demonstrated by shifts to the right of the dose-response curve), followed by a loss of maximal response.*

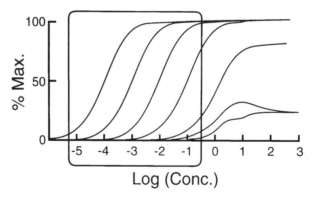

FIGURE 7-9. *Window of responsiveness for a biologic preparation. Within a certain concentration range, agonists may produce a selective response. When this range is exceeded, secondary effects are observed that can affect the slope, threshold, and maximal asymptote of the dose-response curve.*

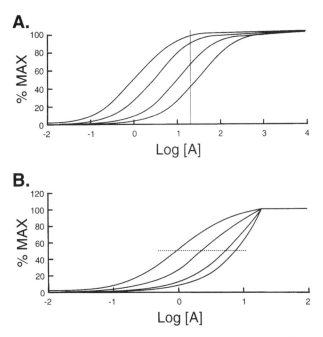

FIGURE 7-10. *A change in shape of the dose-response curve indicates secondary effect. A. A series of dose-response curves to an agonist shifted to the right by the presence of increasing concentrations of antagonist. The vertical line indicates a region beyond which the biologic preparation produces another response to the agonist via a secondary mechanism not sensitive to the antagonist. B. The resulting dose-response curves reflect this change in response pattern in the region of high concentration. The sigmoidal shape is lost.*

can be used as a measure of drug effect. However, the basic principle of biologic amplification—complications with respect to response self-cancellation notwithstanding—suggests that cellular systems with an end-organ response readout can be very valuable. For example, though different cell types produce different responses to drugs, depending on their makeup and location, all cells regulate respiration as a basic biologic function. One result of this regulation is the extrusion of hydrogen ion. Thus, as the metabolism of a cell changes, so too does the rate at which the cell extrudes hydrogen ion in efforts to maintain pH balance (Fig 7-11); this can be measured as a response. The advantage of this system is that it is common to all cells, and therefore, any culture of cells theoretically can yield a biologic response under these conditions (2).

There are other functional assays that rely on special cells to indicate changes in second-messenger levels. One of these is the frog melanophore. These cells disperse pigmentation with increased cyclic AMP levels and concentrate pigment in response to various agonists. Therefore, changes in pigmentation, which can be viewed directly by light transmission, can be used to monitor changes in cytosolic levels of mediators which, in turn, can be con-

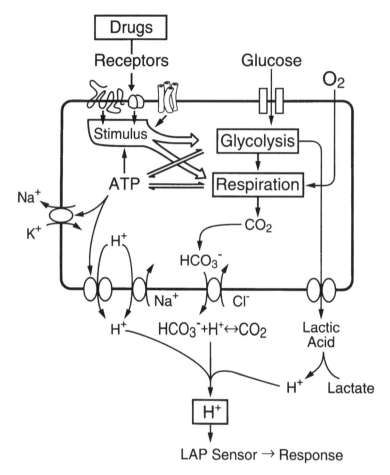

FIGURE 7-11. *The control of hydrogen ion release by cells as an indicator of metabolic cellular activity. Any change in cellular function, such as that produced by drug-receptor interaction, affects cytosolic adenosine triphosphate concentrations, glycolysis, and respiration. These processes affect cellular carbon dioxide, the control of which leads to changes in the hydrogen ion secretion. Thus, hydrogen ion output becomes a sensitive indicator of cellular metabolism and drug-receptor interaction.*

trolled by receptors. Therefore, drugs that alter levels of cyclic AMP or other second messengers produce changes in pigmentation, a functional response that can be quantified and used to measure drug effect. This methodology can be made considerably more powerful by using these cells as hosts for genetically expressed human receptors. Under such circumstances, receptors can be introduced into a response-indicating cell (see Chapter 2), and a functional assay for that receptor can be constructed.

Still another type of functional assay can be made by introducing "reporter" substances into cells. These change their state with changing levels of cytosolic messenger. For example, fluorescent proteins, which produce a phosphorescence with increased levels of cyclic AMP, can be introduced into cells. When a drug activates receptors to elevate cyclic AMP, the cells fluoresce, a response that can be measured photometrically. Another variant of this approach introduces calcium-sensitive proteins, such as aequorin, which produce light on cytosolic elevation of Ca^{++}.

7.4 MEASUREMENT OF DRUG RESPONSE

In general, drug response is measured as a change in state (this can be a rate or a product) from a basal state to some steady state (or state at an arbitrary time point) obtained in the presence of drug. There are basically two reference points needed to assess the status of the drug response: the *basal state* in the absence of drug and the *maximal response* the system is able to produce in response to the same stimulus. The basal state is always observed, but the maximal response can be problematic. There are a number of transforms used for drug-dependent variables (such as response); these are shown in Figure 7-12A. Clearly, the first is the raw response. Use of this parameter is

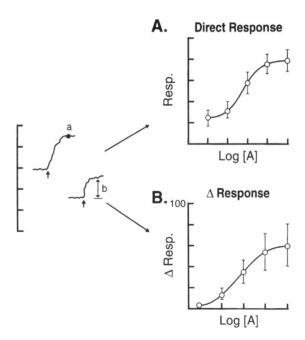

FIGURE 7-12. *Two methods of depicting the response to drugs. A. Direct response. The plateau response of the drug (point a) is plotted directly, with no correction for the resting baseline tissue response present before the drug is added. B. Delta response. The difference between the basal response and the steady state plateau response is plotted as a function of log concentration. This corrects for variances in the resting rates of activity of different biologic preparations.*

hazardous because it does not compensate for the magnitude of either reference point (i.e., the basal state or the maximum response). Therefore, variation in the magnitude of these is reflected as variation in the drug response, with a concomitant loss in accuracy. Another most common technique is to use the difference in system state in the absence and presence of drug (ΔResponse in Fig 7-12B). This has the advantage of cancelling differences in basal effects.

Once a response indicator has been chosen, there are a number of methods to express it for quantification. Clearly, the most straightforward would be to use the actual response readout. The major problem with this approach is that the variances in the basal activities of more than one preparation are added into the magnitude of the drug response, thereby adding error. The effects of response variation can be minimized by replication. Figure 7-13 shows the biologic activity of a hypothetical system. The basal activity, sensitivity to drugs, and maximum response capability of drugs have been subjected to random noise by a computer for 40 different preparations (seven concentrations of drug, resulting in 280 random responses). The resulting responses were randomly mixed further such that there was no correlation between responses to successive doses. Under these circumstances, the scenario whereby only one response to one concentration could be measured for a given preparation was produced thereby allowing construction of dose-response curves from a number of random preparations.

As expected, if only one dose-response curve is assembled in such a way, there is a high degree of variability and a poor representation of the mean

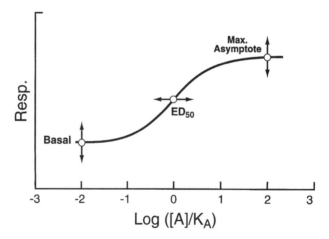

FIGURE 7-13. *Regions of error in dose-response curves from biologic preparations. A hypothetical model was computer-constructed of 40 dose-response curves from 40 preparations of varying basal activities, sensitivities to the agonist, and maximal response capability. Seven drug concentrations were simulated to yield a total database of 280 responses. These were randomized for the calculations shown in Figures 7-14 to 7-17.*

response (Fig 7-14A). If this process is repeated, however, and the resulting dose-response curves averaged, a more accurate representation of the true curve is obtained. Figure 7-14B shows the means of successive curves obtained in this manner. It can be seen that at this level of variability, a reasonably accurate curve is obtained with the mean of 15 to 20 replications. The standard error of the mean of the responses distributes along the concentration in a homogeneous fashion, referred to as a *homeoscedastic error* (Fig 7-14C).

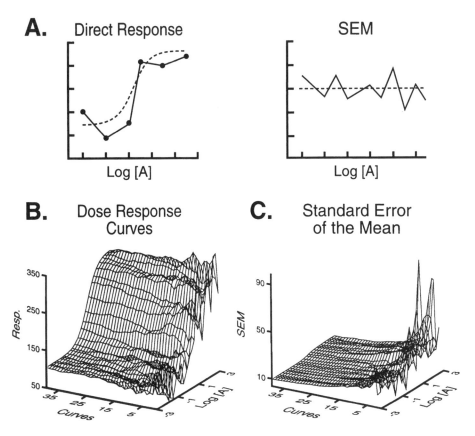

FIGURE 7-14. *Direct response plotted as a function of log concentration. A. Seven random responses from the pool were chosen and plotted as a single dose-response curve (the seven responses come from different biologic preparations). This simulates a condition in which only one response per preparation can be obtained. Dose-response curves necessarily must be constructed with data from different tissues. The standard error for mean (SEM) curves made in this way does not depend on the dose of drug. B. Forty such dose-response curves chosen by computer and sequentially averaged (i.e., the fifth curve is the mean of five curves, the tenth curve is the mean of ten curves, etc.). By the time 20 curves are averaged, a relatively smooth curve results. C. The standard error decreases with the number of curves averaged.*

As discussed previously, a reduction in the error of response measurements can be achieved by eliminating the variances in basal responses by subtracting the basal response from the drug-induced response. This uses only the increased biologic activity to the drug (Fig 7-15A). Figure 7-15B shows the results of this transform on the randomly generated data from Figure 7-14B. Clearly, since the basal response is artificially reduced to zero, the variation in the curves is minimal at the threshold and increases with the dose of the drug. This introduces a heterogeneity in the error, increasing as the magnitude of the response increases (heteroscedastic error; Fig 7-15C). The transform does reduce the error with fewer replications.

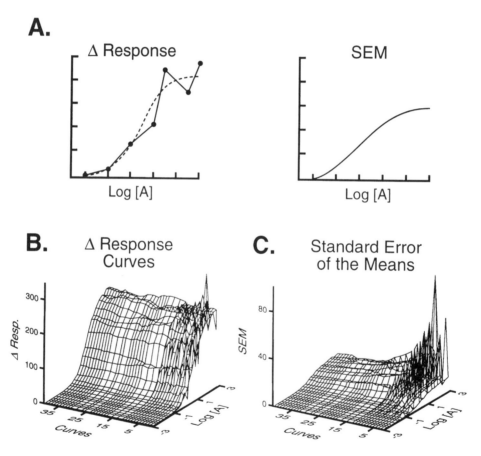

FIGURE 7-15. *Delta response calculated from the dataset shown in Figure 7-14. A. The difference between basal and plateau drug response is plotted as a function of log concentration. Errors range from zero at the threshold of the dose-response curve to maximal values at the maximal asymptote. B. Forty simulated curves (as for Fig 7-14B). C. Standard errors of the means (SEM) for the averaged curves. Note the dependence of error on concentration and inordinately high values of error at the maximal asymptote when few dose-response curves are averaged.*

An alternative method for reducing the impact of baseline variations is to express the response as a percentage of the basal level. Figure 7-16A shows the effects of this transform on the randomly generated data. In general, the trends with this approach are similar to those obtained with subtraction of the basal response (Fig 7-15A), but the variation can be much greater (Fig 7-16B). This is because the percentage increase of a preparation with a low basal tone will be considerably greater than the response in a preparation with a high level of basal tone. Averaging such datasets results in a high degree of variability. In general, the errors from such a transform are extremely heteroscedastic, being greatest at the maximal asymptote (Fig 7-16C).

By far the best estimates of drug response are obtained in preparations in which the basal effects are neutralized (by subtraction of basal response) and the variability of the maximal capability of the system is eliminated. This is

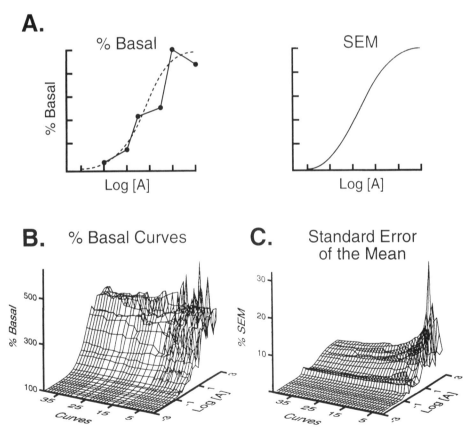

FIGURE 7-16. *The response is presented as a percentage of the basal response. A. The standard error of the mean (SEM) depends on the concentration of drug (as for Δ response). B. The averaged 40 curves indicate wide variation, and a smooth curve is not evident even after 40 averaged dose-response curves. C. The standard error depends on concentration and is high.*

done by measuring the maximal response of the particular preparation and expressing the response of interest as a percentage of that maximum (Fig 7-17A). Clearly, this is possible in only those preparations that allow the measurement of more than one response to drug. Figure 7-17B shows the means of random percentage maximal responses (i.e., each of the single randomly obtained responses was recalculated as a percentage of the maximum in that particular preparation). As can be seen from this figure, a stable mean response is obtained after fewer replications. The error assumes a Boltzmann-like distribution, being 0 at the threshold and maximum, due to the fact that these are set to 0 and 100 respectively (Fig 7-17C). Therefore, the

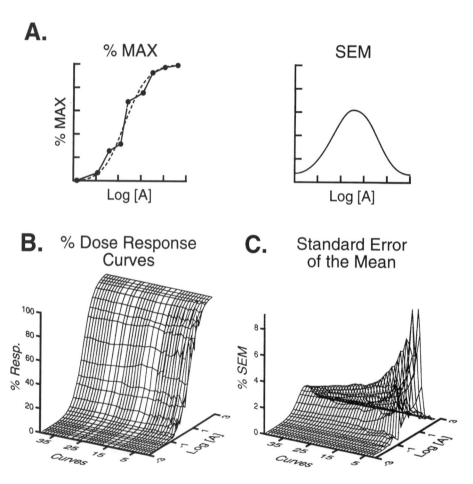

FIGURE 7-17. *The Δ response is calculated as a percentage of the maximal Δ response. A. The distribution of the standard error of the mean (SEM) is bell-shaped, being low at the threshold and maximal asymptote. B. Averaged curves do not change appreciably with respect to location or shape. C. The standard error is highest at the 50% effective concentration (EC$_{50}$).*

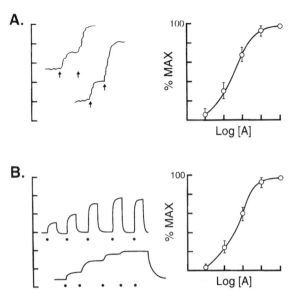

FIGURE 7-18. *Sequential and cumulative dose-response curves. A. The measurement of a response to a drug followed by the measurement of the maximal response in that same preparation. In these circumstances, the response to each drug is scaled for the particular biologic preparation. B. Complete dose-response curve obtained in a single biologic preparation. Some tissues can be repeatedly challenged with drug to obtain a full dose-response curve. Other preparations give sustained responses such that a cumulative effect of the drug can be observed to yield a dose-response curve.*

only variation observed is in the sensitivity of the preparations (the 50% effective concentration [EC_{50}] values).

An even better estimate of the biologic response to a drug can be obtained from preparations that allow the determination of a complete dose-response curve (Fig 7-18). Such valuable systems are the mainstay of receptor pharmacology in that many of them allow for repeated dose-response curves with little change in sensitivity. Under these circumstances, null methods can be used to delineate distinct drug-receptor effects.

7.5 RESPONSE AND TEMPORAL EFFECTS

There basically are three ways to measure response: steady-state rate of response, steady-state product, and cumulative product. Of these, the first two refer to situations whereby sufficient equilibration time theoretically can be allotted between the drug and the receptor (and the accompanying response readout processes) to ignore temporal constraints. Ideally, the temporal behavior of response can be visualized to ensure that a steady state has been attained—that is, the response can be measured in real time. In contrast, the cumulative product response is completely time-dependent and thus requires an arbitrary equilibration time that serves to minimize temporal effects on observed drug activity.

7.5.1 Experiments in Real Time

It is much more convenient and accurate to conduct experiments in real time, and to obtain the dependent variables at the time they are generated. The alternative is, in essence, to take a snapshot of the experiment, arbitrarily stop the reaction, and assess the product: (the experiment is done in "stop-time"). Although this latter approach obviously is flawed, there are many instances in which it is necessary (*vide infra*). This type of experiment has the disadvantage that the time point chosen may not reflect the drug receptor reaction accurately. This becomes more of a problem with more complex responses (i.e., functional cellular responses), because biochemical reactions all have kinetic properties and the product depends on, not only the quantity of reactants but also the rate at which those reactants interact. The advantages of experiments done in real time can be illustrated with a simple example.

Suppose that a given biologic response consists of the production of a biochemical second messenger within a cell. Most second-messenger levels (i.e., cyclic AMP, inositol phosphates, Ca^{++}) are tightly regulated within the cytosol. For example, phosphodiesterase enzymes degrade cyclic AMP, thereby preventing the attainment of extraordinarily high, and therefore toxic, levels. Such controls also allow for temporal responsiveness; that is, cells respond to the initial stimulus but, when this is removed, they quickly revert to their basal state. Therefore, many response systems possess such a control system that removes the second messenger and, therefore, also the response. This oversimplification already exhibits a great deal of complexity in that there are, minimally, eight control parameters that can vary in such a system, four for the production of the second messenger and the same four for the degradatory system. These are: 1)the maximal capacity of the system, 2)the sensitivity of the system, 3)the rate of onset for the reaction, and 4)the rate of offset of the reaction. Varying combinations of these parameters can produce widely differing response characteristics. One example is given here.

Assume that the cell has a system with a given sensitivity to produce a positive response (positive sigmoidal dose-response curve, designated response 2 in Fig 7-19A) and a 66% capability to degrade the second messenger with a 10-fold greater sensitivity (inverted dose-response curve, designated response 1 in Fig 7-19A). If the rates of these two opposing reactions were equal, then clearly no increase in the amount of second messenger would occur. However, a system wherein the production of second messenger is very fast and the degradation, although occurring at a lower concentration, is very much slower, will produce a complex pattern of responses. The time courses

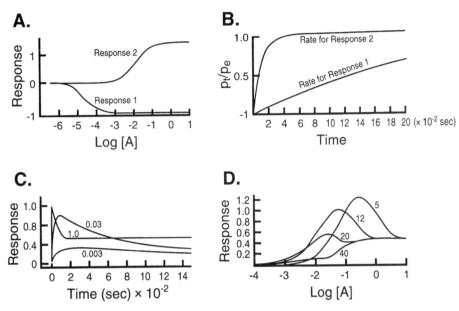

FIGURE 7-19. *Complex responses with differing temporal sensitivity. A. The preparation produces two opposing responses to an agonist. Response 1 is more sensitive and causes a decrease in cellular metabolism. Response 2 is of lower sensitivity and causes an increased cellular metabolism. B. The rate of production of response 2 is considerably higher than the rate of production of response 1. C. The production of three responses with three different concentrations of agonist; effect of equilibration time with agonist. A low concentration (0.003) increases monotonically, a higher concentration (0.03) increases to a maximum and then fades, and the highest dose (1.0) produces a sharp peak and then fades sharply. D. Dose-response curves to the agonist taken at four different times of exposure to the agonist. Note the complete change in threshold, slope, shape, and maximal asymptote of the curves (to the same agonist) taken at different times.*

for the two reactions are shown in Figure 7-19B; they were chosen deliberately so that the most sensitive reaction (response 1) was the slower one.

Under these circumstances, the time course for the production of response will vary with concentration because of the differing sensitivity of the two responses to substrate. Figure 7-19C shows the time course for three concentrations of a drug that stimulates the production of the second messenger. Such complexity raises immediate practical problems in that the peak response occurs at *different* time points for different concentrations. In these circumstances, the resulting dose-response curves to a complete set of drug concentrations are complex and change shape with time (see Fig 7-19D).

A more comprehensive picture of the interplay between time and concentration in such a system can be seen in three dimensions. Figure 7-20A shows a series of dose-response curves to the agonist, obtained at different time points as a surface. Some idea of the stop-time dose-response curves can be

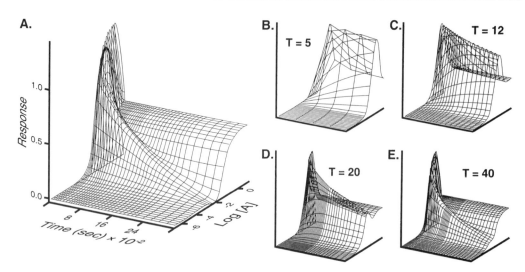

FIGURE 7-20. *Dose-response curves for the system described in Figure 7-19 taken at various times. A. The evolution of the changes in shape of the dose-response curve when it is measured at various time points. B–E. Expanded views of portions of A indicating the resulting curve after 5 min (B), 12 min (C), 20 min (D) and 40 min(E).*

seen in Figure7-20B,C, D, and E, in which the reactions are stopped at 5, 12, 20 and 40 minutes from time 0. These frozen time points are the same as those shown in Figure 7-20D. This example illustrates the possible effects of time on the apparent potency of drugs or sensitivity of biologic systems. Often these effects are unavoidable, and some arbitrary time point must be chosen for analysis. However, the ability to measure the reaction in real time allows observation of the most stable periods for analysis and can avoid artifacts of equilibration time.

7.5.2 Experiments in Stop-Time

The alternative to working in real time is to allow reactions to continue for a set time period, to stop them and to view the results. As discussed previously, the inherent disadvantage of not being able to the view steady state (i.e., to stop the reaction when no further change is taking place) is obvious. However, there are numerous instances in which this is necessary. For example, in radioligand-binding experiments, the amount of radioactive ligand that is bound to the receptor must be measured, and this requires that the radioactivity be quantified, which in turn takes time. Thus, the binding reaction must be stopped at a given time point before a determination of how far the reaction has gone can be made.

An illustration of a stop-time reaction of two drugs with differing kinetics is shown in Figure 7-21. Figure 7-21A illustrates the rate of receptor activation

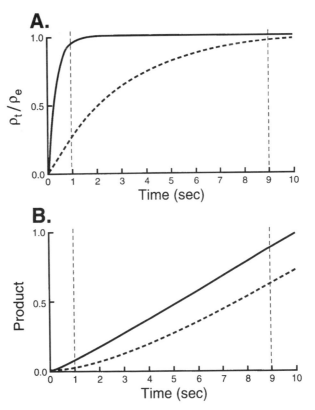

FIGURE 7-21. *Cumulative biochemical product as a stop-time response. A. The rate of production of a biochemical product to two equiactive agonists of differing rates of onset. The amount of product formed is the area under the respective curves. B. The area under the curve plotted as the response with time. The vertical lines indicate two stopping points for the reaction. The early time point severely underestimates the response to the slower agonist. This is reflected in the differentially low amount of biochemical product as a fraction of that made by the faster agonist. This difference is considerably lessened by stopping the reaction at the later time point.*

by the drugs; the agonist represented by the solid line has a considerably faster rate of onset. The fractional rate of activation for a first-order rate of onset can be modeled by the following equation:

$$\frac{\rho_t}{\rho_e} = 1 - e^{-(k([A] + K_A))t} \qquad [7.3]$$

where the rate of receptor occupation at time t is ρ_t and equilibrium activation is ρ_e. The rate of onset is denoted by k, and the equilibrium dissociation constant of the drug for the receptor is K_A.

The two vertical dotted lines in Figure 7-21A indicate two different stop times; the furthest to the left clearly is before a steady state is reached, whereas the line at the right is at a time when nearly complete activation has occurred. In a stop-time reaction in which the product of the receptor activation is measured (e.g., the production of a cellular metabolite), the amount of product is given by the area under the curves shown in Figure 7-21A. This is expressed as the integral of Equation 7.3:

$$\frac{\text{Area}_t}{\text{Area}_e} = t + \frac{e^{-(k([A]+K_A))t}}{k([A]/K_A + 1)} - \frac{1}{k([A]/K_A + 1)} \qquad [7.4]$$

The area under the curves shown in Fig 7-21A as a function of time for the two agonists is shown in Fig 7-21B with the accompanying two reaction stop-time points. What is noteworthy about the reaction product lines is the distinct curvature at early time points. This corresponds to the shortage of production due to incomplete rate of onset: Little reaction product is formed when the receptor activation has not yet reached steady state. This deficit is more pronounced with drugs of slower onset (note the dotted line corresponding to the slower agonist); therefore, an error is introduced into the amount of product measurement due to the difference in rates of activation. This error becomes less important with longer equilibration times (note the percentage relative response of both drugs at the two stop-times). In general, the period for accumulating of biochemical products in stop-time experiments should err on the side of being longer than needed to minimize errors due to differences in drugs' rates of onset.

7.6 SYNOPSIS

The following ideas were presented in this chapter:

- Drugs and drug receptors can be studied either with biochemical binding or by the observation of system function in response to drugs; there are respective strengths and weaknesses to both approaches.

- In general, function studies address partial receptor populations, whereas binding studies involve whole populations. With function, extraordinary selectivity can be achieved by virtue of the fact that only small selective receptor occupancies are required.

- In binding studies, systems should be maximized to achieve maximum specific binding (low levels of nonspecific binding), adequate equilibration times to reach steady state, and the lowest possible aberration of ligand concentration by binding to receptors.

- Biologic preparations generally have a window of stability with an initial unstable period (for equilibration and recovery from trauma) and period of declining function (due to inadequacy of in vitro methods to sustain them). It is tacitly assumed in all experimentation that the system sensitivity has not changed.

■ Changes in the shape of dose-response curves during receptor manipulation (i.e., addition of antagonist) can be indicative of secondary effects of agonists.

■ There are a number of methods to express response to drugs. Indices of raw tissue function can be obscured by variances in basal tissue function. Transforms such as delta response (response minus basal response) reduce basal effects but can skew the distribution of error.

■ The best indicator of tissue sensitivity and drug response is obtained when a response can be measured along with a measure of the maximal response that can be elicited in the tissue. The delta response expressed as a percentage of this maximal delta normalizes data for different tissues.

■ Experiments in real time are preferable to those in stop-time because the kinetics of response production can be viewed. Experiments in stop-time can produce errors in comparisons between drugs with different rates of onset. This can be minimized by longer equilibration times.

REFERENCES

1. Limbird LE. Cell Surface Receptors: A short course on theory and methods. Boston: Martinus Nijhoff, 1985.
2. McConnell HM, Owicki JC, Parce JW, et al. The cytosensor microphysiometer: biological applications of silicon technology. Science 1992;257:1906–1912.

FURTHER READING

Armitage P. Statistical methods in medical research. Oxford: Blackwell, 1971.
Finney DJ. Experimental design and its statistical basis. Chicago: University of Chicago Free Press, 1955.
Riggs DS. The mathematical approach to physiological problems. Baltimore: Williams and Wilkins, 1963.
Tallarida RJ, Murray RG. Manual of pharmacologic calculations with computer programs. Berlin: Springer-Verlag, 1979.
Waud DR. Analysis of dose-response relationships. In: Narahashi TL, Bianchi CP, eds. Advances in general and cellular pharmacology. New York:Plenum Press, 1976.

Drug Antagonism

THE MOST POWERFUL techniques for determining molecular mechanisms of receptor function involve the antagonism of receptor response. Antagonism can be classified by the effects of an antagonist on the dose-response curve (section 8.1). The most useful form of antagonism, in terms of defining receptor function, is competitive antagonism, because competitive antagonists produce mathematically predictable effects on agonist response (section 8.2). The single most useful tool in this regard is the Schild regression, which also can be used to define nonequilibrium steady states in receptor systems (section 8.2.1), heterogeneous receptor populations (section 8.2.2), and receptor antagonism occurring concomitantly with other effects (resultant analysis; section 8.3.3). Sections 8.3 and 8.4 discuss receptor blockade by partial agonists and irreversible antagonists, respectively. The complex effects of noncompetitive antagonists are discussed in section 8.5. These ideas are reviewed in the synopsis (section 8.6).

8.1 TYPES OF ANTAGONISM

The general meaning of the term *drug antagonism* suggests that one drug interferes with the action of another. There are a number of ways this can occur. In the first, the drug acts on another receptor on the host, and the product of that reaction interferes with the action of the primary drug. This is referred to as *physiologic* (or *functional*) *antagonism*. Although this has been modeled in the past in operational terms, it is difficult to divine useful data from such interactions, mainly because of the multitude of mechanisms possible and the dependence of the conclusions on the specific model chosen to make the analysis. The remaining two ways in which one drug can interfere with the actions of another, however, have been studied quantitatively, and from these a paradigm for the quantification of drug and system properties has been obtained.

The way that one chooses the theoretical framework to work in for a given set of drug-receptor interactions is by observation of the effects of the antagonist on dose-response curves to the agonists. The classic pharmacologist Sir John Gaddum proposed two terms to define operationally the type of antagonism a given ligand could induce on the effects of a given agonist (1). The first described a drug which blocked the effects of an agonist but did not depress the maximal response to that agonist. This type of antagonist was labeled a *surmountable antagonist*. This term was chosen because it connoted the fact that, even though the antagonist necessarily caused an increase in the dose of agonist to be used to achieve an equal response to that obtained in the absence of the antagonist, with enough agonist, the maximal response to the agonist could be achieved (Fig 8-1A). In contrast, the term *insurmountable antagonist* was coined for a drug that, when present, precluded the attainment of the maximal response to that agonist no matter what the dose of agonist (Fig 8-1B). As mentioned previously, these terms are descriptive and simply serve to characterize observed antagonism operationally. However, it will be seen that this is the first step in linking the observed pattern of antagonism to a molecular mechanism. As a preface to how this occurs, a discussion of the molecular mechanisms of antagonism is useful.

The discerning factor in the study of antagonism is the interaction of the two drugs on a common receptor. This can occur in one of two ways: either the drugs can compete for interaction at the same site or they can interact with different sites on the receptor such that the receptor reacts to the most prevalent signal and modifies its behavior toward the host accordingly (2). The first type of interaction is termed *competitive* (*syntopic*), whereas the latter (interaction at separate sites on the receptor molecule) is termed *allotopic*. Also, the term *competitive* should be qualified temporally.

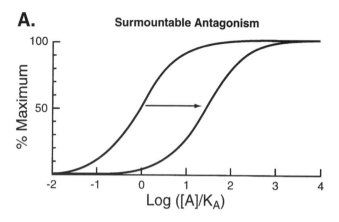

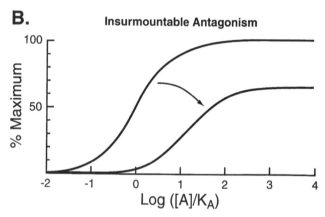

FIGURE 8-1. *Dose-response curves to an agonist depicting surmountable and insurmountable antago-nism. A. Surmountable antagonism is denoted by a parallel shift of the dose-response curve with no diminution of maximal response. B. Insurmountable antagonism may or may not produce a shift to the right of the location parameters of the dose-response curve but is characterized by a decrease in the maximal response.*

A classic competitive antagonist is reversible in that it has kinetics of onset and offset comparable with those of the agonist. Therefore, as stated in Chapter 1, a competitive reversible antagonist can bind to a receptor that is temporarily vacated by an agonist (due to thermal energization) but, the reverse also can occur; that is, the antagonist can vacate the receptor because of thermal effects and allow an agonist molecule to replace it. In contrast, a type of one-way competition can occur between an irreversible antagonist and an agonist. In this scenario, the antagonist binds irreversibly to the receptor (either because of a chemical reaction with part of the receptor [*vide infra*] or because the kinetics of offset are so slow that the reaction, in the time frame of the agonist reaction, is so slow as to be considered essentially irreversible), but because the binding site is the same as that required by the agonist, the interaction still is considered chemically competitive.

In molecular terms, certain patterns of effects on dose-response curves can be imprinted by competitive and allotopic antagonists. Competitive antagonists generally produce a parallel shift to the right of the dose-response curve with no depression of maximum. Obviously, there are constraints on the limit to which the shift can occur (e.g., secondary effects of the agonist, toxic effects, solubility limits) but, theoretically, a competitive antagonist can produce an infinite shift to the right of the dose-response curve to an agonist. In contrast, allotopic antagonists can have multiple effects on dose-response curves. The effects could be identical, within a range of concentrations, to those of a competitive antagonist. Alternatively, an allotopic antagonist could preclude agonist activation of receptors and produce a depression of the maximal response (i.e., produce insurmountable antagonism). The effects of a simple reversible competitive antagonist can be differentiated from those of an allotopic antagonist by examination of the increasing concentrations of each on the dose-response curve. The effects of an allotopic antagonist result from the saturation of a limited number of binding sites, thus, the magnitude of the dextral displacement of the curve will converge to a constant value (obtained when all the allotopic binding sites are occupied). In contrast, as stated previously, the dextral displacement produced by a competitive antagonist theoretically is infinite as it is caused by the competition between the agonist and the antagonist for a population of binding sites (Fig 8-2).

Finally, an irreversible antagonist (but one that may or may not compete with the agonist binding site) can produce either surmountable or insurmountable antagonism. Which of these is observed depends on the response being measured and the degree of amplification imposed on the signal (*vide infra*). An irreversible antagonist produces a decrease in the number of operative receptors; thus, a depression of the receptor-occupancy curve would be observed on treatment with an irreversible antagonist. However, if tissue response is the readout for the drug effect and the tissue amplifies the receptor events such that only a submaximal receptor occupancy by agonist can produce maximal tissue response (i.e., there is receptor reserve capacity), then the irreversible inhibition of a population of receptors will cause a parallel shift to the right of the dose-response curve to the agonist. Under these circumstances, the steady state effects will formally resemble those of a simple reversible competitive antagonist. However, temporal examination of the effects of each can be used to differentiate them. The effects of a reversible competitive antagonist will appear with a first-order rate of onset and come to steady state with increasing equilibration time. In contrast, an irreversible antagonist will progressively alkylate receptors with increasing equilibration time and not come to a steady state (Fig 8-3).

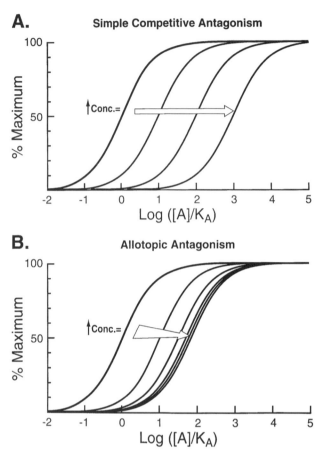

FIGURE 8-2. *The effects of increasing concentrations of simple competitive and allotopic antagonists. A. Simple competitive antagonists produce dose-related shifts to the right of dose-response curves with theoretically no limiting effect. B. Allotopic antagonists produce an effect that comes to a limit when all of the allotopic receptor sites are saturated by the antagonist.*

8.2 COMPETITIVE ANTAGONISM

By far the most valuable type of drug-receptor interaction for the characterization of a biologic receptor is competitive antagonism. This is because there are simple relationships between agonist effect and the concentrations of antagonist that allow both testing of the mathematic model on which the molecular interactions are based and calculation of the chemical constant of interaction between the antagonist and the receptor. *The nature of this constant allows it to be transferable across all systems containing the receptor; hence, it becomes an operational fingerprint for the receptor.* This, in turn, can be used to study the receptor in a variety of environments and to compare it to other new systems and thereby possibly classify new receptors.

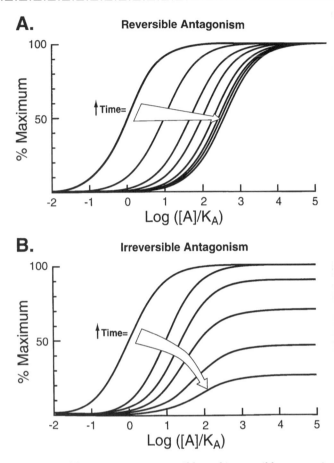

FIGURE 8-3. *Effects of increasing equilibration time on reversible and irreversible antagonists. A. Reversible antagonists show increasing effect with increasing equilibration time toward an equilibrium value. Once equilibrium is established, further equilibration time has no further effect on the antagonism. B. In contrast, the effects of an irreversible antagonist increase with increasing equilibration time with no steady state (except when the antagonist is chemically depleted from the medium).*

The central equation from which all other relationships are derived is the Gaddum equation (3):

$$\rho_A = \frac{[A]/K_A}{[A]/K_A + [B]/K_B + 1} \qquad [8.1]$$

where the fractional receptor occupancy for the agonist A is given by ρ_A, the concentration of the antagonist is denoted by $[B]$, and the equilibrium dissociation constants of the agonist-receptor and antagonist-receptor complexes, respectively, are given by K_A and K_B. It is worth inspecting Equation 8.1 as a tool to compare receptor occupancies by an agonist in the presence and

absence of a competitive antagonist. For example, in the absence of an antagonist ($[B] = 0$), at a concentration of agonist equal to the K_A, 50% of the
receptors are occupied by the agonist ($\rho_A = 0.5$). However, in the presence of
an added concentration of antagonist equal to the K_B, the agonist receptor
occupancy decreases to 33% (Fig 8-4). As discussed in Chapter 1, both the
agonist and the antagonist occupy and vacate the receptor in concomitant
stochastic processes. Normally, the agonist binds to receptors not already
occupied by itself according to the magnitude of the K_A and its concentration.
However, in the presence of an antagonist that competes for the same binding
site, the agonist will have a statistically lower chance of finding an unoccupied
receptor; therefore, the agonist occupancy decreases (i.e., receptor antagonism results).

There is another feature of Equation 8.1 worth noting—namely, that the
same receptor occupancy can again be achieved by the agonist, even in the
presence of an antagonist. Thus, if the agonist concentration is doubled (i.e.,
if it is increased from $[A] = K_A$ to $[A] = 2 \times K_A$), then a receptor occupancy
of 50% ($\rho_A = 0.5$) again can be achieved. In this sense, *competitive* means that
both drugs compete for receptor occupancy and, by increasing concentrations, either can dominate (see Fig 8-4).

This competition occurs throughout the concentration range for the
agonist and results in a definitive pattern for the effects of an agonist in the
presence of a competitive antagonist. If Equation 8.1 were used to calculate a

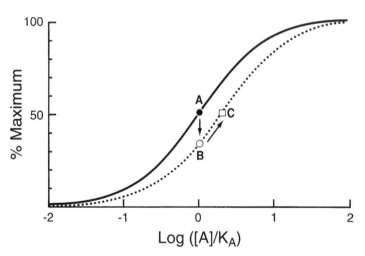

FIGURE 8-4. *Simple competitive antagonism. A concentration of antagonist is present that produces a
twofold shift in the dose-response curve to the agonist. Thus, a 50% effective concentration (EC_{50}) response (point A) is reduced to point B in the presence of the antagonist.
However, a doubling of the concentration of agonist brings the response back to the
original level (point C). The negative logarithm of the competitive antagonist producing
such an effect is referred to as the pA_2.*

series of dose-response curves to the agonist in the absence and presence of varying concentrations of antagonist, the pattern shown in Figure 8-5A would be seen. Thus, *a competitive antagonist produces parallel shifts to the right of the dose-response curve to an agonist with no diminution of maximal response to the agonist.* Moreover, there is a strict formal relationship between the concentration of antagonist present at the receptor (as a multiple of the K_A) and the resulting shift to the right of the dose-response curve produced. This relationship is one of the most important in receptor pharmacology and can be used to characterize receptors, drugs, and the assumptions of drug equilibrium and

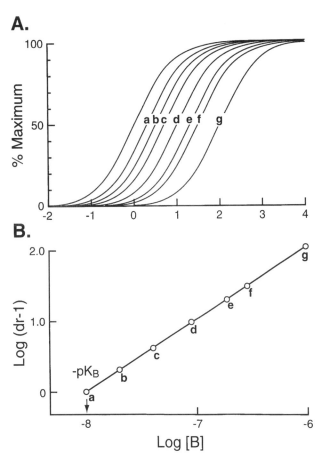

FIGURE 8-5. *Schild analysis. A. Increasing concentrations of a simple competitive antagonist produce increasing shifts to the right of the agonist dose-response curve. B. The shifts shown in A [calculated as the logarithm of equiactive agonist dose-ratios (dr)minus 1] are plotted as a function of the logarithms of the concentrations of antagonist that produced them, to construct a linear regression. If simple competitive antagonism is operable, the regression should be linear, have a slope of unity, and an intercept corresponding to the pK_B ($-Log\ K_B$).*

selectivity. The relationship was derived by the pharmacologist Heinz Schild and its use is termed *Schild analysis* (4):

$$dr = \frac{[B]}{K_B} - 1 \qquad [8.2]$$

Where *dr* is the dose ratio for equieffective concentrations of agonist in the presence of the antagonist and absence of the antagonist. Thus, a dose ratio of 2 means that in the presence of the antagonist, the concentration of the agonist must be doubled to achieve the same response as that obtained before addition of the antagonist (see Fig 8-4). It can be seen from Equation 8.2 that a concentration of antagonist that produces a dose-ratio of 2 will be equal to the K_B. *In general, when a competitive antagonist is present in the receptor compartment in a concentration equal to its K_B, it will produce a twofold shift to the right of an agonist dose-response curve.*

Equation 8.2 embodies the concept of increasing shift to the right of agonist dose-response curves with increasing antagonist concentration: That is, the more antagonist present to compete for free receptor, the less probability exists for occupation of the receptor by agonist. To increase this probability, the concentration of agonist must be increased (i.e., higher dose ratio).

The relationship between the dose ratio (an experimentally observed parameter), the concentration of antagonist (an experimentally controlled parameter), and the equilibrium dissociation constant of the antagonist-receptor complex (K_B) is an important aspect of Equation 8.2. This latter parameter is extremely valuable as it is a chemical constant unique for every antagonist-receptor combination. Schild recognized this and formatted Equation 8.2 into a logarithmic metameter:

$$\text{Log } (dr - 1) = \text{Log } [B] - \text{Log } K_B \qquad [8.3]$$

Known as the *Schild equation*, this has broad implications in receptor pharmacology. A regression of a succession of dose ratios [plotted as Log $(dr - 1)$] on the logarithm of the concentrations of antagonist that produced them should yield a straight line with a slope of unity and an *x*-intercept equal to *Log K_B* (see Fig 8-5B).

The estimation of K_B values is a mainstay of receptor pharmacology and variations of the Gaddum equation can be used to estimate this value. The most comprehensive approach is by Schild analysis as this affords a test for competitiveness. Specifically, a truly competitive antagonist should produce parallel dextral displacements of dose-response curves that result in a linear Schild regression with a slope of unity. A full Schild analysis is composed of a dataset consisting of a full dose-response curve to the agonist obtained in the absence of the antagonist and in the presence of a range of concentrations of antagonist. The resulting dose ratios are plotted as Log $(dr - 1)$ values on the logarithms of the molar concentrations of antagonist. If this is observed, then there is presumptive evidence to assume that the resulting intercept is a measure of the K_B. If this is not observed (i.e., if the regression is not linear or is linear with a slope different from unity), then either the antagonist is not competitive or other factors are obscuring the actions of the antagonist (*vide infra*). In this case, the concentration of antagonist that produces a twofold shift to the right of an agonist dose-response curve cannot be assumed to equal the K_B. It then is referred to as the pA_2, *an empiric constant that is the negative molar concentration of antagonist observed to produce a two-fold shift to the right of a dose-response curve.* By definition, the pK_B is always the pA_2 whereas the converse is not necessarily true: A pA_2 may not be the true pK_B.

Though competitive antagonists should produce parallel shifts of the dose-response curves under ideal conditions, this may not be evident from the data sample (Fig 8-6A). Under such circumstances, there are statistical methods available (see Chapter 9) to test for parallelism and, should the data satisfy the assumption, parallel lines can be fit simultaneously to the complete dataset (Fig 8-6B). This is preferred because it allows for the calculation of dose ratios, the magnitude of which do not depend on the level of response.

There are instances when a full Schild analysis is not possible or practical. In these cases, competitive antagonism is assumed and either partial dose-response curves or variations of the Gaddum equation are used to measure the K_B (Fig 8-7A). For example, it may not be practical to obtain full dose-response curves to the agonist in vivo. In this situation, a common maximal response is assumed, and the dose ratios are used to calculate the pK_B (Fig 8-7B). Note that two important assumptions are made—namely, that the antagonist is competitive and that the maximal response is unchanged as the dose-response curve is shifted to the right. Keeping in mind that these assumptions may seriously limit the interpretation of the data, the parallel curves fit to the model curves can be used to calculate dose ratios (Fig 8-7C).

Another common approach is to fix the concentration of agonist and vary the concentration of antagonist. As shown in Figure 8-8A, a concentration [A] of agonist is chosen that produces a measurable response. The response produced by this concentration of agonist in the presence of a range of concentrations of antagonist is shown as well; there is predicted shifting to the right of the agonist dose-response curve. As can be seen from this figure, the magnitude of the response to the concentration [A] decreases with increasing concentrations of antagonist. If this response is plotted as a function of the logarithm of the concentration of antagonist, the curve shown in Figure 8-8B is obtained. This is a useful method for determining the active concentration range of the antagonist: Region I in this figure is below the threshold for antagonism, II is the region of antagonism, and III is complete antagonism.

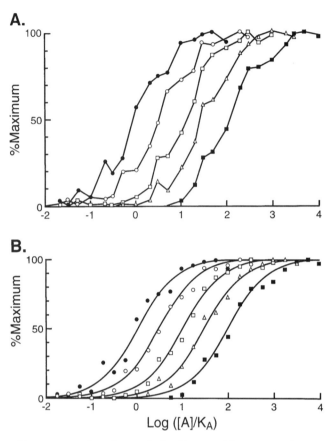

FIGURE 8-6. *Fit of curves with common slope for analysis of competitive antagonism. A. A series of dose-response curves from single estimates of response. Data points joined with straight lines. B. Same data with a computer fit of logistic function curves of common slope. In these circumstances, dose ratios become independent of the level of response used to measure them.*

Data in regions I and III are not useful because a measure of the potency of the antagonist cannot be gained in these regions.

These types of curves furnish an important empiric measure of antagonist potency; that is, the inhibitor concentration that produces 50% inhibition of response, or the IC_{50}. The empiric nature of this parameter stems from the fact that its magnitude depends on the concentration of agonist used for the reference response. If a low dose of agonist is used, then low doses of antagonist are required to block it; the IC_{50} will reflect this and be a low concentration. If a higher dose of agonist is used, then higher concentrations of antagonist will be required and the IC_{50} value will be correspondingly higher, as shown in Figure 8-9.

This raises a practical question: Does the fact that an antagonist produces no effect on a given agonist response mean that it is inactive (present in a

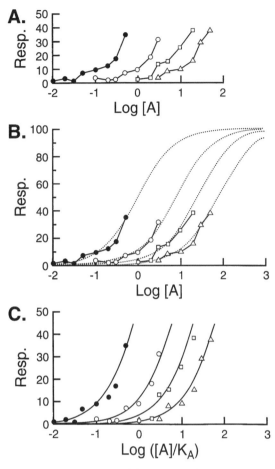

FIGURE 8-7. *Use of partial datasets to estimate competitive antagonist potency. A. A series of partial dose-response curves in a system in which it is not possible to measure the maximal response. B. Computer fit of logistic curves with common slope and maximum to the partial datasets. C. The same data as shown in A with the common slope partial logistic functions.*

concentration below its threshold for receptor occupancy), or does it mean that the agonist concentration is so high that there is not enough antagonist present to produce measurable antagonism? An obvious approach to solving this problem, is to track antagonism of a submaximal concentration of agonist. Also, there is reason to choose as low a level of response as possible to block with the antagonist. A rearrangement of the Gaddum equation (Equation 8.1) shows a potentially useful relationship between the molecular constant K_B and the IC_{50} for the agonist signal. The following equation can be derived:

$$\frac{[IC_{50}]}{K_B} = \frac{[A]}{K_A} + 1$$

[8.4]

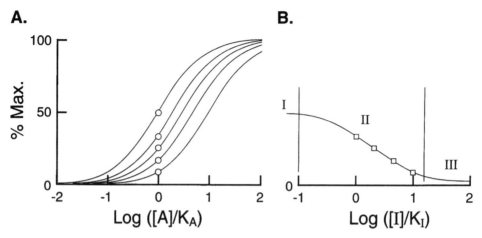

FIGURE 8-8. *Estimation of antagonist potency by varying antagonist concentration at constant agonist concentration. A. The effects of increasing concentrations of antagonist on the dose-response curve to an agonist. The circles indicate the effects of the antagonist on a single concentration of agonist [the 50% effective concentration (EC_{50})]. B. The same response points denoted by circles in A plotted as a function of the concentration of antagonist used to produce the antagonism. In region I, the concentration of antagonist is subthreshold and no effect on the agonist response is seen. Response is sensitive to the antagonist in region II. In region III, the effects of the antagonist are supramaximal, and no information about antagonist potency can be obtained.*

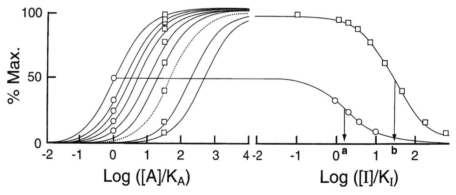

FIGURE 8-9. *Dependence of the 50% inhibitor concentration (IC_{50}) on the concentration of agonist (or radioligand) being antagonized. The circles refer to the effects of an antagonist on the 50% effective concentration (EC_{50}) of stimulating drug (agonist or radioligand). The IC_{50} for the antagonist blocking this amount of stimulation is denoted by point a. In contrast, the blockade of a concentration of stimulating drug producing 90% maximal response (squares) requires higher concentrations of antagonist. The IC_{50} for this level of stimulation is denoted by point b.*

From Equation 8.4 it can be seen that if a concentration of agonist or in the case of radioligand-binding studies, a concentration of radioligand (see Chapter 7) is chosen that is substantially lower than the K_A, then $[A]/K_A \to 0$ and the $IC_{50} \to K_B$. Figure 8-10 shows the relationship between the concentration of the agonist (or radioligand) used in the analysis and the concentration of antagonist needed to produce a 50% inhibition of the stimulus (IC_{50}). From this figure it can be seen that the K_B value approximates the IC_{50} until the concentration of agonist approaches the equilibrium dissociation constant of the agonist-receptor complex (K_A). At higher concentrations of agonist, a correction according to Equation 8.4 must be made to calculate the K_B from the IC_{50}. It is important to quantify antagonist potency in terms of K_B because this constant is transferable between assays (being independent of the concentration of agonist being blocked).

In general, all these latter methods assume competitive antagonism under ideal conditions and thus have an intrinsic weakness. By far the better approach is to use Schild analysis, which has built-in tests of these assumptions and thereby yields a confidence level for the resulting K_B estimate. An important distinction should be made between the pA_2 and the pK_B obtained from Schild analysis. The theoretic basis of the method assumes simple competitive antagonism, which dictates that a slope of unity for the regression must be obtained. In practice, the sampling of data may not be sufficient to satisfy this criterion (i.e., the experimental slope may not equal unity because of random error in the sample). In this case, the intercept of the Schild regression is the pA_2 value

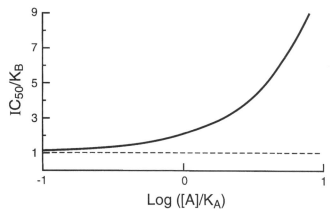

FIGURE 8-10. *The effect of stimulation level (either agonist concentration or radioligand concentration) on the 50% inhibitory concentration (IC_{50}). At levels of stimulation below the equilibrium dissociation constant for half-maximal effect (either half-maximal receptor occupancy or half maximal response), the IC_{50} approximates the true K_B. However, as this stimulation intensity is exceeded, the IC_{50} deviates from the K_B and a correction according to Equation 8.4 must be made.*

and not the pK_B. However, if statistical analysis of the data indicates that the 95% confidence limits of the slope include unity (i.e., there is a 95% chance that the slope is truly unity), *then the dataset should be recalculated to a Schild equation of slope unity.* This implies that if enough experimental data points were to be collected, the slope of the experimental curve would be unity and that any differences would be due to random error. The reason for constraining a slope to unity is that an intercept from a slope not equal to unity has no meaning in molecular terms. Unless the criteria of Schild analysis are satisfied, the resulting estimate does not conform to the model of simple competitive antagonism. However, if it can be shown that the data sample is a valid representation of the population and statistically satisfies the requirements of Schild analysis, then the recalculated regression can be used to determine the molecular constant pK_B. Figure 8-11A shows a theoretic dataset for Schild analysis. The calculated slope of the regression is 1.14, but the 95% confidence limits of this slope include unity. Therefore, the regression has been recalculated to a line of slope unity (solid line) and the resulting intercept used as the pK_B. This particular case has been chosen to illustrate the importance of where the dataset resides in the concentration range of the antagonist. Because data points were obtained at values both lower and higher than the pK_B, the differences in the estimate made by the two regressions are extremely small (i.e., the pK_B is obtained by interpolation). However, if the same type of data were to be obtained with concentrations producing shifts in the dose-response curves of 10 or greater, then the difference between the experimental and the constrained slope leads to an appreciable difference in the estimate of the intercept (Fig

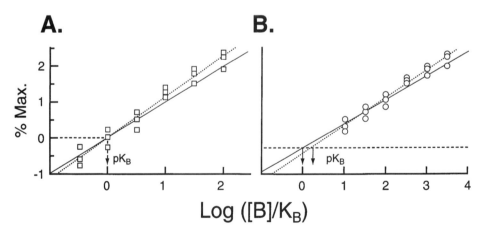

FIGURE 8-11. *The effect of concentration range of data for Schild analysis. A. The data spans the concentration range containing the pK_B. The interpolated pK_B is relatively insensitive to variances in data and slope. B. The regression is calculated from data comprising dose ratios (dr) greater than 10, and the pK_B is extrapolated. In this case, the pK_B estimate depends more on the variance in the data and slope.*

8-11B; pK_B obtained by extrapolation). In general, it is best to obtain data that allow interpolation, rather than extrapolation, of the pK_B.

8.2.1 Detection of Nonequilibrium Steady States

In addition to the measurement of antagonist potency, Schild analysisis is also useful for uncovering possible nonequilibrium steady states in drug-receptor experiments. Theoretically, an infinite number of dose ratios can be obtained for an agonist in the presence of an antagonist. However, there is a practical limit to the concentrations of agonist that can be used in a biologic system to achieve response. Beyond that practical limit, other factors obscure the production of response thereby causing deviation from the predictions of the Schild equation. Figure 8-12A shows a theoretic series of shifts to the right of

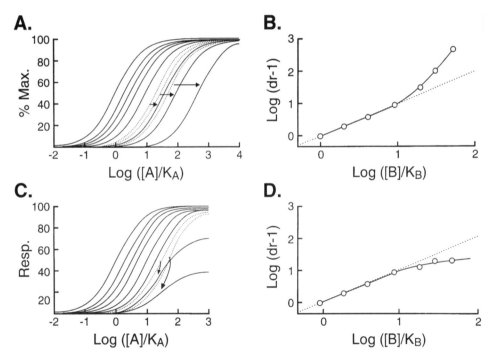

FIGURE 8-12. *Recognition of deviation from equilibrium behavior with Schild regressions. A. Shifts of a dose-response curve to an agonist produced by a simple competitive antagonist. These can be used to calculate a Schild regression. B. Schild regression calculated from the data shown in A. As the dose-response curve is moved into regions of concentration that produce a secondary effect (in this case, a decrease in responsiveness), the corresponding shifts of the curve deviate from those predicted by the single action of simple competitive antagonism. The Schild regression reflects this with a curvilinear deviation from ideal behavior. C. Data similar to A except that higher concentrations of agonist produce depressed maximal responsiveness and a potentiation of sensitivity to the agonist. D. The resulting Schild regression (data from C) shows the region of deviation from ideal behavior.*

the dose-response curves into a concentration range where toxic effects are encountered. As this occurs, the simple relationship between *dr* and antagonist concentration breaks down because factors other than simple competitive antagonism are operative in the biologic system. The result is a nonlinearity of the Schild regression as the dose ratios progress into the concentrations of agonist at which toxic effects are seen (Fig 8-12B). Similarly, such nonspecific effects can cause decreases in the effects of antagonists or depressions of the maxima of dose-response curves (Fig 8-12C). Schild regressions are sensitive indicators of where such effects begin (Fig 8-12D). These simulations illustrate one of the most practical applications of Schild analysis—namely, definition of the size of drug selectivity windows.

The Schild equation defines the interaction of two drugs at a receptor and adherence to that definition requires that no other factors change during the analysis. Therefore, if simple competitive antagonism of an agonist occurs within a given concentration range of antagonist to produce a 300-hundred fold shift of the dose-response curve ($dr = 300$), then it can be assumed that over that concentration range the agonist produces a *selective* activation of the receptor. The linear portion of the Schild regression defines a selectivity window for the process of a two-drug interaction at the receptor. Therefore, any perturbation of this delicate balance will be detected by the quantitative relationship between response and the reactants (i.e., Schild analysis can detect deviation from equilibrium). The slope of the Schild regression is a sensitive indicator of the relationship between the concentration of drugs (both agonist and antagonist) in the receptor compartment and the receptors. If a simple relationship between these exists that adheres to Langmuirian kinetics, then the regression will be linear with a slope of unity. This will be referred to as *ideal behavior*. There are a number of nonequilibrium conditions that can cause the slope of the Schild regression to deviate from unity.

Obviously, if secondary actions of the antagonist or the agonist produce displacement of the agonist dose-response curves greater than those produced by competitive antagonism, the augmented dose ratios will be indicated by an increase in the slope of the Schild regression (i.e., see Fig 8-12B). In addition, at least two nonequilibrium but chemically defined conditions can cause a steeper slope for the Schild regression. The first is a lack of temporal equilibrium for a first-order rate of onset for the antagonist; that is, the antagonist has not been allowed enough time to equilibrate completely with the receptors. For a first-order process, the concentration of the antagonist determines the rate of onset; therefore, lower concentrations require a longer time of equilibration than do higher concentrations. If the time of the equilibration is insufficient, then the Schild regression will reflect this condition as an inequality of antagonistic effect; in other words, the lower concentrations of antagonist that are not yet equilibrated with the receptors will be less affected than higher concentrations of antagonist (5). The result will be a differential in the dose ratios between low and high concentrations of antagonist that yields a steep slope for the Schild regression (Fig 8-13A).

A second cause of steep slopes for Schild regressions is the saturable removal of the antagonist from the receptor compartment. For example, rabbits have a natural enzyme able to degrade the muscarinic antagonist atropine; therefore, low concentrations of this antagonist do not equilibrate with receptors in the receptor compartment due to degradation. Under these conditions, the concentrations of atropine in the receptor compartment are much lower than those added to the medium and the dose ratios for these low concentrations are underestimated. However, higher concentrations of atropine saturate this enzymatic degradation; consequently, the concentration added to the medium equals that in the receptor compartment and the dose-ratios increase proportionately to those predicted by the Gaddum equation. The result of these types of processes are Schild regressions greater than unity (see Fig 8-13B).

There also are conditions that are indicated by Schild regression slopes of less than unity. Clearly, as indicated earlier, if the antagonist potentiates agonist response or the agonist produces a secondary response in some range

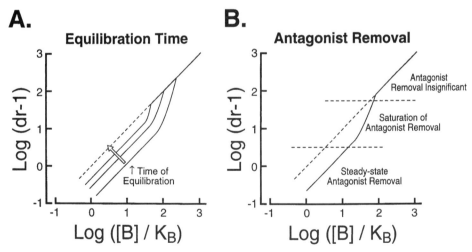

FIGURE 8-13. *Experimental nonequilibrium conditions that produce Schild regressions with slopes greater than unity. A. Inadequate time of equilibration produces a condition whereby the effects of lower doses of antagonist are underestimated compared to those of higher doses. The result is a nonlinear regression with portions of slope greater than unity. Increased equilibration time corrects the error. B. If the antagonist is removed from the receptor compartment by a saturable process (e.g., enzymatic degradation), then increasing the concentration of antagonist to one at which the removal process is saturated (and thus is negated) produces an increase in the concentration of antagonist at the receptor. The result is an increased dose ratio in this region and a steep Schild regression.*

of concentrations, then the dose ratios will diminish with a corresponding decrease in the slope of the Schild regression (6). However, a decrease in slope also can indicate some chemically well-defined nonequilibrium conditions. Specifically, if the agonist is removed from the receptor compartment by a degradation or uptake process (i.e., see Chapter 5), and if the concentration range for agonism is driven toward concentrations of agonist that saturate this removal process, then a dissimulation between the concentration of agonist added to the medium and that producing response will be observed. At low dose ratios of the antagonist, where the concentrations of agonist are too low to saturate removal, there will be a deficit between the concentrations of agonist added to the medium and those in the receptor compartment. If this were to remain constant throughout the Schild analysis, then no perturbation of dose ratios (and, therefore, the Schild slope) will occur. If, however, the removal process were to be saturated as the concentrations of agonist are increased (due to receptor blockade), then more of the agonist being added to the medium will reach the receptor compartment and, in essence, the agonist response will be "potentiated" with a resulting diminution in dose ratio. The result is a decrease in the slope of the Schild regression (Fig 8-14A).

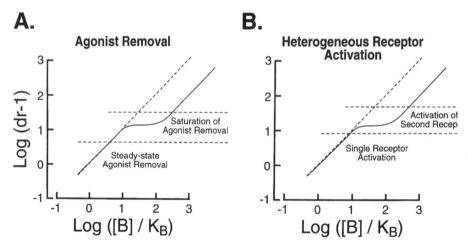

FIGURE 8-14. *Experimental nonequilibrium conditions that produce Schild regression with slopes of less than unity. A. If the agonist is removed from the receptor by a saturable process, then moving the dose-response curve into regions of concentration that saturate agonist removal will produce an incremental increase in the concentration of agonist at the receptor. This will produce an incremental increase in response, with a resulting decrease in dose ratio, which is indicated by a nonlinear Schild regression with portions of slope less than unity. B. If the agonist activates a secondary receptor system (that is not sensitive to the antagonist) at higher doses, then as the dose-response curve to the agonist is moved into this concentration region, an added response will be produced. This will be reflected in a reduced dose ratio and a nonlinear Schild regression with portions of slope less than unity.*

This is a common experimental phenomenon and therefore a useful method to *detect* removal processes for agonists in receptor systems.

Another common mechanism for decreases in Schild regression slopes is activation of secondary receptor populations. Under these circumstances, the agonist produces proportionally greater response in a selected region of the concentration range, which can result in a decrease in dose ratio if the antagonist is not of equal or greater potency than an antagonist of the secondary receptor population (Fig 8-14B).

8.2.2 Detection of Heterogeneous Receptor Populations

The detection of heterogeneous receptor populations in receptor systems can be achieved by use of Schild analysis. Two approaches are available. The first is to observe nonlinearity and differences in slope of the Schild regression as the agonist activates the secondary receptor population, as discussed previously (see Fig 8-14B). The second is to repeat the Schild analysis with different agonists for the same receptor. The rationale for this approach is the idea that different agonists probably would not have identical affinities and efficacies for the two receptor types, and so the contribution of the two populations for each agonist will differ. Under these circumstances, a selective antagonist will have differing abilities to block these mixed agonists. For example, consider the effects of two agonists: One, agonist *A*, primarily produces response by activation of the receptor most sensitive to the antagonist, and the other, agonist B, generates a large proportion of response from another receptor less sensitive to the antagonist. Under these circumstances, the overall response to agonist *A* will be blocked to a greater extent by the antagonist than will the response to agonist *B*. The divergence in antagonist potency augurs the involvement of more than one receptor to the overall response to the agonists (Fig 8-15).

8.2.3 Pharmacologic Resultant Analysis

A technique developed by Sir James Black and colleagues makes use of the additivity of dose ratios to quantify the potency of antagonists that have other properties that might obscure their primary effect (7). For example, consider a competitive antagonist that also blocks the cyclic AMP degradatory enzyme phosphodiesterase and thus elevates basal cellular activity. The result of these two activities would be antagonism (shift to the right of the dose-response curve) and an elevation of baseline function (inhibition of phosphodiesterase; Fig 8-16A). If the agonist being used was involved in cyclic AMP metabolism, then a potentiation of the agonist effect also might be observed. The observed effects of the antagonist would not be suitable for normal Schild analysis for the measurement of pK_B (see Fig 8-16B). However, the combination of this complex antagonist (to be termed the *test antagonist*) and another

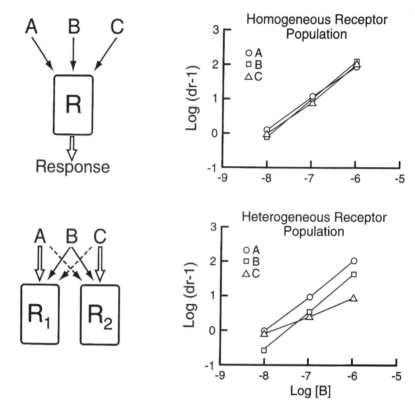

FIGURE 8-15. *The detection of multiple receptor populations with Schild analysis. (Top) All three agonists (A,B,C) activate a single receptor. The resulting Schild regressions for all three agonists for a given antagonist will be identical. (Lower) Two receptor populations are present in the tissue and the three agonists have varying activities at each of them. The antagonist has varying potency on the two receptor populations as well, leading to different sensitivities of the three agonists to the antagonist. This results in three different Schild regressions for the same antagonist when measured with the three different agonists. This behavior is indicative of a heterogeneous receptor population.*

known simple competitive antagonist (termed the *reference antagonist*) can be analyzed. Specifically, the receptor preparation is treated with a given concentration of test antagonist, and the response to the agonist is determined. This curve will be the result of a complex function of primary antagonism and secondary effects (in this example, potentiation due to phosphodiesterase blockade). Then, the reference antagonist is added, and the response to the agonist again is determined. Under these circumstances, the secondary effects of the test antagonist can be nullified as both curves were determined in the presence of the same concentration of test antagonist (see Fig 8-16C). Therefore, the difference between the first and second curve will be due solely to the effects of added reference antagonist. Because the concentration and pK_B of the reference antagonist are known, the contribution of this antagonist to the

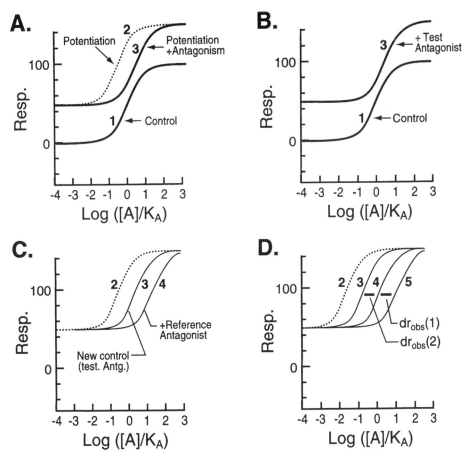

FIGURE 8-16. *Pharmacologic resultant analysis. A. The effects of the test antagonist on a dose-response curve to an agonist (denoted control curve 1). The test antagonist has two properties— namely, that of potentiation of both basal and agonist-induced response (curve 2) and receptor antagonism (addition of this property produces curve 3). B. The observed effect of the test antagonist on the control response. The control curve is shifted to the left with an increased basal effect, making Schild analysis impossible. C. The addition of the reference antagonist to the system already equilibrated with the test antagonist is to produce further receptor antagonism (curve 4). No effects on the basal response are produced by the reference antagonist. D. Further additions of the reference antagonist to the system produces further shifts to the right of the dose-response curve (curve 5). These shifts [$dr_{obs}(1)$, $d_{obs}(2)$] can be used to estimate the already present receptor antagonism produced by the test antagonist and allow the estimation of the pK_B for this drug.*

observed dose ratio can be determined. The observed dose ratio will be given by the Schild equation:

$$dr_{obs} = 1 + ([B]_{test}/K_b + [B]_{ref}/K_B)$$

[8.5]

By obtaining a number of dose-response curves to the agonist in the presence of a range of concentrations of reference antagonist, a Schild regression for the reference antagonist can be obtained that gives an apparent pK_B for the reference antagonist which is in error by the contribution made by the test antagonist. Repetition of this analysis in the presence of difference concentrations of test antagonist permits these apparent pK_B estimates for the reference antagonist to be used to calculate the relationship between the contribution to the observed dose ratios produced by the test antagonist and the corresponding concentration of test antagonist. Because the contributing dose ratios and corresponding $[B]_{test}$ are known, the K_{Btest} can be calculated. The receptor antagonist properties of drugs with multiple properties can be determined using this technique (Fig 8-16D).

8.3 ANTAGONISM BY PARTIAL AGONISTS

A special class of antagonist comprises partial agonists which are drugs that produce a low level of agonist response resulting from binding to the receptor. The partial agonist produces shifts to the right of dose-response curves to full agonists (in the manner of a simple competitive antagonist), but this effect will be overlaid on an intrinsic agonist response to the partial agonist itself. Figure 8-17 shows a dose-response-curve to a partial agonist and the resulting effects of various concentrations of the partial agonist on a dose-response curve to the full agonist.

8.4 IRREVERSIBLE ANTAGONISM

One class of drugs blocks receptors irreversibly, by forming covalent bonds with the protein of receptors, and they cannot be removed by washing with drug-free media. One example of a large group of such drugs is β-halo-alkylamines (Fig 8-18A), which form reactive aziridinium ions in aqueous medium and go on to alkylate a number of sites on proteins. Another class of alkylating agent utilizes activation by light to form a reactive species. Thus, photoactive azides interact reversibly with receptors until exposed to ultraviolet light (Fig 8-18B). With photoactivation, they form a reactive species that goes on to alkylate the receptor protein. In general, two variables associated with alkylating agents must be considered in their use: concentration and time of equilibration. Unlike reversible drugs, an irreversible reaction will continue until the reactants (either receptor or drug) are depleted. Therefore, the time of exposure of a receptor preparation to an alkylating drug must be carefully controlled if a selective alkylation of receptor protein is required. Figure 8-3B shows the effects of continuing time of exposure of a receptor system to an alkylating agent.

Irreversible drugs attain some measure of selectivity by virtue of a selective affinity of the receptor (over other proteins)— so-called affinity labeling. The

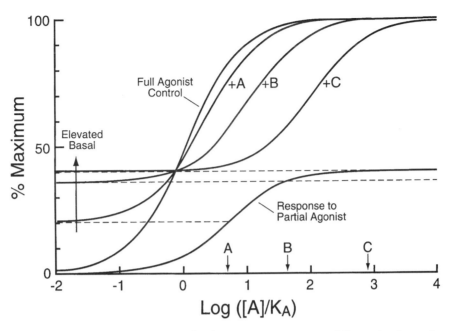

FIGURE 8-17. *The effects of a partial agonist on the dose-response curve to a full agonist. Increasing concentrations of the partial agonist, produce an increase in the baseline response. The dose-response curve to the agonist is shifted to the right by the presence of the partial agonist and this curve is superimposed on the elevated baseline. Concentration A of the partial agonist produces half the maximal response to the partial agonist and occupies 50% of the receptors. This concentration produces a twofold shift to the right of the agonist curve. Concentration B occupies 90% of the receptors and produces a 10-fold shift of the curve. Concentration C occupies 99% of the receptors and produces a 100-fold shift of the full agonist curve.*

alkylating drug, by virtue of its particular chemical structure, concentrates near the receptor in higher concentrations than at any other protein in the preparation. If the drug is chemically reactive (such as β-haloalkylamines), the colocalization with the receptor will lead to preferential alkylation of the receptor. If the activation can be controlled externally (i.e., photoalkylation), then the drug can be equilibrated with the preparation to achieve maximum colocalization, and then photoactivation can form the alkyl bond. Because the alkylation process is of shorter duration, it usually is more selective. Irreversible drugs have a number of uses. For example, if the drug is distinguishable (i.e., radioactive or fluorescent), then it can be used to label the receptor for biochemical isolation.

Another feature of irreversible alkylation is the selective elimination of drug response by knockout of receptors. Figure 8-19A shows the effects of an alkylating agent on the receptor occupation of an agonist. As the receptors are occluded, the maximal receptor occupancy is reduced. However, for some high-efficacy agonists that can produce maximal response in a receptor

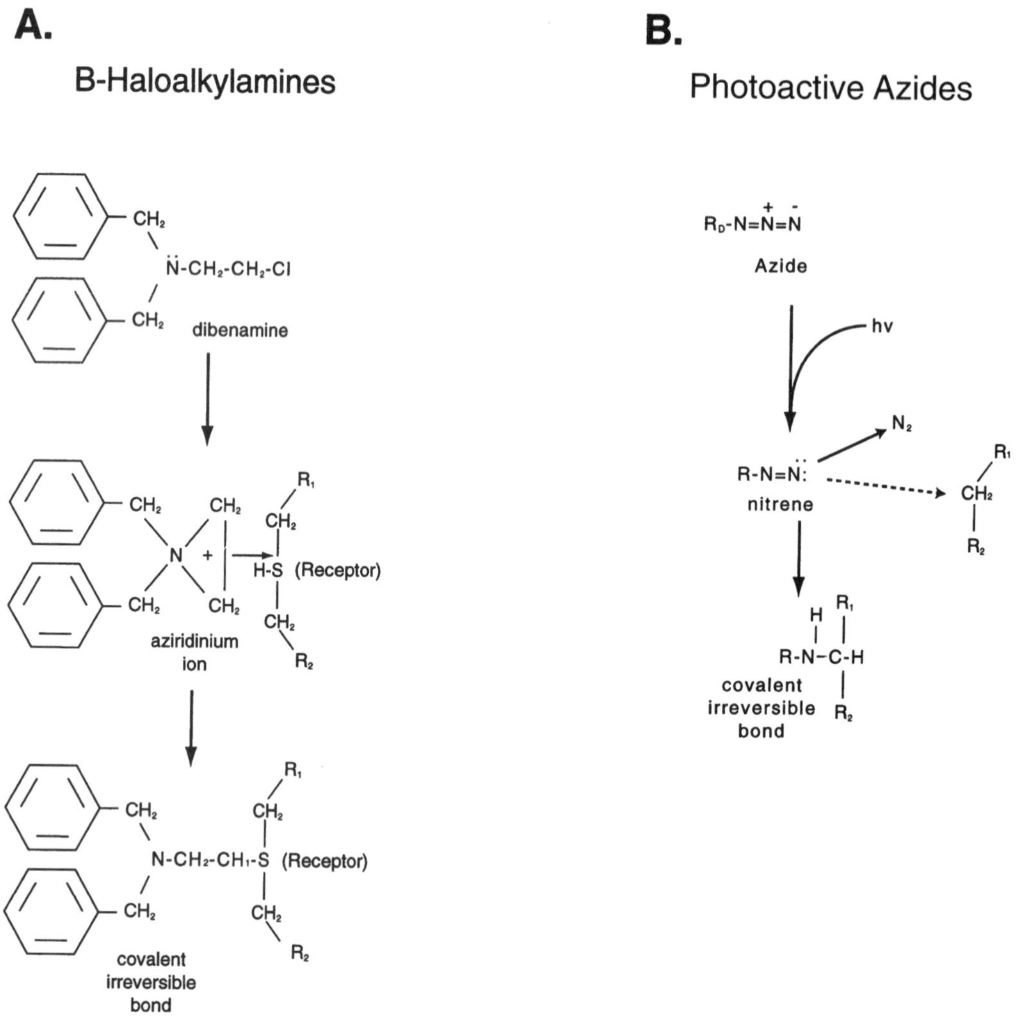

A.

B-Haloalkylamines

B.

Photoactive Azides

FIGURE 8-18. *Chemical mechanisms of alkylation of receptor protein by irreversible antagonists. A. β-Haloalkylamines produce a highly reactive aziridinium ion, which then goes on to insert into a variety of chemical bonds. B. Photoactive azides produce a reactive center on exposure to light, which then goes on to insert into a number of chemical bonds.*

preparation by activation of only a few receptors (receptor reserve), alkylation of a portion of the receptors will not reduce the maximal response if the portion is below the spare capacity of the system (Fig 8-19B). Further alkylation beyond this critical fraction (the fraction required to produce maximal response to the agonist) finally will produce a reduction in the maximal response. Thus, the sequential alkylation of receptors and observation of the resulting effects on the responses to different agonists can be used to determine the relative contribution of efficacy and affinity to the potency of an agonist. Figure 8-19A shows the effects of alkylation on a weak agonist (i.e.,

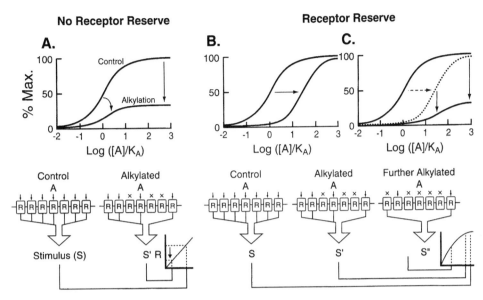

FIGURE 8-19. *The effects of irreversible antagonism in different receptor systems. A. Alkylation of a portion of the receptor population in a system in which the maximum signal requires activation of the complete receptor population. Under these circumstances, a depression of the maximal asymptote of the curve is observed. B. In a system with receptor reserve in which the maximal signal can be produced by activation of only a portion of the receptor population, alkylation of some of the receptors will produce a shift to the right of the dose-response curve with no corresponding decrease in the maximal asymptote. Further alkylation beyond the receptor reserve level produces depression of the maximum.*

low efficacy), whereas Figure 8-19B shows the effects of the same treatment with alkylating agent on responses to a highly efficacious agonist.

8.5 NONCOMPETITIVE (ALLOTOPIC) ANTAGONISM

There also are ligands that modify or preclude agonist activation of receptors in a reversible manner; these are referred to as *noncompetitive antagonists* as they can exert their effect by binding to a site different from that required by the agonist. Two aspects of receptor mechanisms need to be discussed for noncompetitive antagonists. The first is the effect of the antagonist on the ability of the agonist to produce response. The simplest mechanism is inactivation of the receptor on binding of the antagonist.

A second consideration is the effect of antagonist binding on the affinity of the agonist. The simplest assumption is that the binding of the antagonist is independent and has no effect on the binding of the agonist. In essence, the noncompetitive antagonist binds to its own site on the receptor and turns it off from signaling to the agonist. This is the simplest model of noncompetitive antagonism and the one used in early formulations of receptor theory for noncompetitive antagonists.

With this model, it can be shown that noncompetitive antagonists have the operational effects of irreversible antagonists in that they reduce the maximal receptor occupancy but they do not bind in an irreversible manner (i.e., their effects can be removed by washing with drug-free media). Therefore, though they may reduce the maximal response to an agonist, they come to an equilibrium state in the same manner as does a competitive antagonist (Fig 8-20A). If the binding of the noncompetitive antagonist precludes

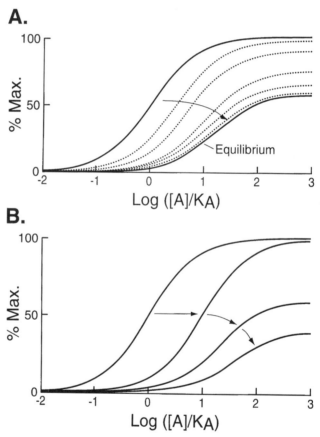

FIGURE 8-20. *The effects of a noncompetitive antagonist. A. Increasing equilibration times for a given concentration of noncompetitive antagonist on the response to an agonist. This particular concentration produces a shift to the right of the dose-response curve and concomitant depression of the maximal response. Unlike irreversible antagonism, the effect comes to equilibrium and further equilibration time with the antagonist does not produce further antagonism. B. Depending on the receptor occupancy and stimulation requirements of the tissue system, noncompetitive antagonists can produce shifts to the right of dose-response curves with no diminution of maximum response or shifts with diminution of maxima.*

agonist activation, then the receptor occupancy for an agonist $[A]$ in the presence of a noncompetitive antagonist $[B]$ is given by the following equation:

$$\rho_A = \frac{[AR]}{[R]} = \frac{[A]}{[A] + K_A} \cdot \left[\frac{1}{(1 + [B]/K_B)} \right] \qquad [8.6]$$

where K_A and K_B refer to the equilibrium dissociation constants of the agonist and antagonist receptor complexes, respectively. It can be seen from this equation that any finite value for $[B]$ will diminish maximal agonist occupancy. Whether this results in a diminution of the maximal response to the agonist again depends on the efficacy of the agonist (see previous discussion on irreversible antagonists). If the agonist is of high efficacy and requires only a small portion of the receptor population to produce maximal response, then a noncompetitive antagonist may produce a parallel shift to the right of the dose-response curve to the agonist (Fig 8-20B). However, if the agonist is of low efficacy and requires maximal receptor occupancy to produce maximal response (or if it is a partial agonist and does not produce the maximal tissue response at full receptor occupancy), then a noncompetitive antagonist will produce a shift to the right and a depression of the maximum of the dose-response curve (see Fig 8-20A).

The preceding discussion describes the simplest case for non-competitive antagonism—namely that of no interaction between the binding sites for the agonist and the antagonist (no cooperation). However, there are cases in which this is not so and in which the binding of one drug (either agonist or antagonist) modifies the receptor's affinity for the other. Under these circumstances, the scheme for receptor binding can be shown as follows:

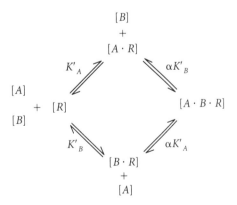

where the agonist is A and the antagonist (also referred to as the *allotopic effector* or *allosteric effector*) is B, K'_A and K'_B are the equilibrium association constants for the ligands and receptors, and α is a multiplicative factor representing the modification of the second ligand's affinity on binding of the first. In such circumstances, the concentration of agonist-receptor complex $[A \cdot R]$ in the presence of a non-competitive antagonist is given by this equation:

$$\frac{[A \cdot R]}{[R_t]} = \rho = \frac{[A]/K_A}{[A]/K_A(1 + \alpha[B]/K_A) + (1 + [B]/K_B)} \qquad [8.7]$$

where K_A and K_B represent equilibrium dissociation constants ($K_A = 1/K'_A$). It can be seen that if $\alpha = 1$ (i.e., there is no interaction between the ligands and the binding of one does not affect the affinity of the other), this equation reduces to Equation 8.6. However, if the binding of one of the drugs affects the affinity of the other (there is an allotopic change in the receptor conformation on binding of one of the drugs), then the observed affinity of the agonist is given thus:

$$\frac{K_{obs}}{K_A} = \frac{(1 + [B]/K_B)}{(1 + \alpha[B]/K_B)} \qquad [8.8]$$

As discussed in Figures 8-2 and 8-3 for allotopic antagonists, the overall change in affinity of the agonist will not increase infinitely but rather will increase to a maximal value (as $[B]/K_B \to \infty$, $K_{obs}/K_A \to 1/\alpha$). The allotopic antagonist will depress maximal response in a manner similar to that shown in Figure 8-20 except that the location parameter (the 50% effective concentration $[EC_{50}]$)of the agonist curve may shift.

The assumption about the signaling capabilities of the receptor when it is occupied by the noncompetitive antagonist raises issues about the depression of the maximal response to the agonist. For example, the receptor may still be able to signal under agonist influence but less efficiently. This can be described by a modifying factor (defined as ξ), which could represent a percentage signaling efficiency of the antagonist bound receptor. Thus, a ξ value of 0.3 would reflect the condition whereby the complex $[A \cdot B \cdot R]$ produced 30% of the signal produced by $[A \cdot R]$. Equation 8.7 can be rewritten to reflect this condition:

$$\frac{[A \cdot R]}{R_t} = \rho = \frac{[A]/K_A(1 + \alpha\xi[B]/K_B)}{[A]/K_A(1 + \alpha[B]/K_A) + (1 + [B]/K_B)} \qquad [8.9]$$

This equation is very similar to Equation 8.7 except that the depression of the maximal response to the agonist is less than if the receptor completely fails to signal when bound by the antagonist.

The point of this type of modeling is to show that numerous mechanisms can produce noncompetitive antagonism and that the effect of noncompetitive antagonists can be varied in terms of effects on agonist affinity and on the maximal response to the agonist. Therefore, it is difficult, without prior knowledge of the molecular mechanism of the noncompetitive antagonist, to predict the pattern of dose-response curves to be expected from noncompetitive antagonists. Likewise, the effect of noncompetitive antagonists on dose-response curves cannot reliably be used to infer molecular mechanism of antagonism. However, the general behavior of producing depressed dose-response curves that come to equilibrium steady states with increasing equilibration time is common to all these mechanisms and thus can be used to detect noncompetitive, as opposed to simple competitive or irreversible, antagonism.

8.6 SYNOPSIS

The following ideas were presented in this chapter:

- Antagonism can be classified operationally, in terms of the effects on an agonist's dose-response curve, as surmountable or insurmountable.

- Antagonists can be classified also in terms of molecular mechanism as competitive (syntopic; interaction at the same site as the agonist) or allotopic (acting at a site distinct from the agonist site but affecting agonist binding). The two can be distinguished by the limited effects of maximal concentration with allotopic antagonists.

- Antagonists can act reversibly or irreversibly with receptors. These mechanisms can be distinguished by the observation of temporal equilibrium.

- The most useful tool for drug and receptor classification is Schild analysis, which can be used to estimate the equilibrium dissociation constant of competitive antagonist-receptor complexes. This method has built-in mechanisms to ensure adherence to the model of simple competitive antagonism.

- The Schild method also can be used to detect nonequilibrium experimental conditions (agonist and antagonist removal mechanisms, temporal dysequilibrium) and heterogeneous receptor populations.

- Other variations on the Gaddum equation calculate antagonist potency in terms of IC_{50} values. To be of use in molecular terms, these must be adjusted for the strength of stimulus being blocked by the antagonist.

- Pharmacologic resultant analysis is a useful technique for measuring the antagonist potency of drugs with multiple (and obscuring) actions in the biologic system.

- Partial agonists produce agonist response and antagonism of responses to full agonists.

- Irreversible antagonists can alkylate receptor protein, but the equilibration time of the receptor with these agents must be strictly controlled to achieve selectivity.

- Noncompetitive antagonists can produce parallel shifts to the right of agonist dose-response curves or depression of the maximal response. They differ from irreversible antagonists (similar effects are produced) in that a temporal equilibrium is achieved.

REFERENCES

1. Gaddum JH. Theories of drug antagonism. Pharmacol. Rev. 1957;9:211–218.
2. Monod J, Wyman J, Changeux JP. On the nature of allosteric transitions. J. Biol. Chem. 1960;12:88–118.
3. Gaddum JH, 1947. Biological aspects: The antagonism of drugs. Trans. Faraday. Soc. 1943;39:323–333.
4. Arunlakshana O. Schild HO. Some quantitative uses of drug antagonists. Br. J. Pharmacol. 1959;14:48–58.
5. Kenakin TP. Effects of equilibration time on the attainment of equilibrium between antagonists and drug receptors. Eur. J. Pharmacol. 1980;66:295–306.
6. Kenakin TP, Beek D. Self-cancellation of drug properties as a mode of organ selectivity. The antimuscarinic effects of ambenonium. J. Pharmacol. Exp. Ther. 1985;232:732–740.
7. Black JW, Gerskowitch VP, Leff P, Shankley NP. Analysis of competitive antagonism when this property occurs as part of a pharmacological resultant. Br. J. Pharmacol. 1986;89:547–555.

FURTHER READING

Ehlert FJ. Estimation of the affinities of allosteric ligands using radioligand binding and pharmacological null methods. Mol. Pharmacol. 1988;33:187–194.
Kenakin TP, Black JW. The pharmacological classification of practolol and chloropractolol. Mol. Pharmacol. 1978;14:607–623.

Statistical and Biologic Significance

THIS CHAPTER addresses the determination of difference and inference of physiologic consequences from numeric data. Specifically, statistics can be used to determine the magnitude of differences, in relation to the magnitude of the error associated with the measurement. Samples from populations are used (section 9.2) to test hypotheses describing the existence of difference (section 9.3). Samples are characterized by their mean and standard error (section 9.4). A frequently used approach involves the analysis of straight lines as these are predictable (section 9.5). Differences also can be described using population analysis (section 9.6). The availability of high-speed computers has made nonlinear curve fitting, an approach with the advantage of not requiring data transformation, a widely used technique (section 9.7). The involvement of statistical principles in experimental design is discussed in section 9.8. These ideas are reviewed in the synopsis (section 9.9).

9.1 INTRODUCTION

The science of statistics is the study of measures of *dispersion* (error) and *central tendency* (e.g., means). In general, quantitative experiments on drug activity (or system sensitivity) are carried out to collect numeric data. These data then can be subjected to statistical procedures to sift out signal-to-noise ratios (i.e., to help distinguish between a true signal, due to the experimental manipulation, and what would have happened anyway, due to the noise of the system). Moreover, statistical procedures can help determine when two signals are samples from the same or different populations. There are two important pharmacologic consequences to such conclusions. The first leads to conclusions about intrinsic differences between drug-receptor systems (e.g., receptor subtypes, isozymes). The second helps draw conclusions about differences between various drugs and the applicability of data obtained in surrogate systems to the therapeutic arena in humans.

9.2 POPULATIONS AND SAMPLES

A useful concept is one of populations and samples. A population is defined as a very large (nearly infinite) collection of data—for example, all the possible responses of a given cell sample to a drug. It often is not possible and always is impractical to attempt to define the complete population experimentally; therefore, a sample of that population is obtained as a representative of the population. For that sample to be a useful representative, it must be obtained in a random manner. If it is biased, then the conclusions about the population will necessarily be incorrect. For example, in drug-receptor experiments, desensitization of physiologic response is a well-known and frequent event. Thus, when physiologic systems are stimulated, they can begin to lose responsiveness. This can be due to a true receptor inactivation (desensitization) or to a modulatory mechanism in the response machinery (tachyphylaxis). This has the effect of reducing the magnitude of successive drug responses. A frequently observed pattern is shown in Figure 9-1A, in which the degree of tachyphylaxis is linked to the intensity of the stimulation. Thus, low doses of drug producing small responses produce a slower-onset but more sustained response. As the intensity of the stimulation increases, the rate of response and the fade of response increase as well.

If the sample of responses from this tissue, obtained to represent the population of possible responses (i.e., to characterize the tissue responsiveness to the drug), were collected in a sequential manner (i.e., low dose to high dose or, alternatively, high to low dose), then a skewed sample would be collected whereby the desensitizing influence of the previous dose would affect the observed response to the next dose. If a definite order of dosing were used then the imposition of that order would introduce a systematic error into the resulting dataset (see Fig 9-1B). One way to minimize the effects of systematic errors on the sample is to collect the sample in a random manner.

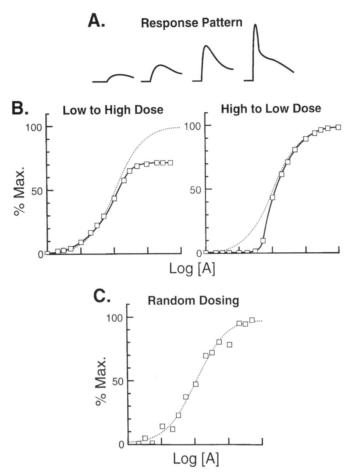

FIGURE 9-1. *Randomization of drug delivery. A. Typical response pattern of an agonist that demon-strates tachyphylaxis. Low-level responses are slower in onset but sustained, whereas higher-level responses are fast but transient. B. If dose-response curves were obtained by sequential delivery of drug—either low-dose to high-dose or high-dose to low-dose—then a systematic error due to the pattern of desensitization may produce a bias in the dose-response curves. Low to high would depress maximal asymptotic responses selec-tively, whereas high to low might selectively desensitize lower-level responses. C. A ran-domization of the dosing tends to distribute the effects tachyphylaxis throughout the dose-response curve.*

In random sampling, the effects of desensitization are more evenly distributed throughout the sampling and thus are minimized. Also, repeated samples will have the same influence throughout; the risk of that one sample will be more heavily influenced by the systematic error than another is eliminated. Among the available randomized procedures for data sample collection is the Latin square, wherein the sequence and magnitude of the doses of drug to be tested are randomized (Fig 9-1C).

9.3 HYPOTHESIS TESTING

As discussed in Chapter 1, hypotheses (ideas that describe a scientific mechanism or entity) cannot be proved correct, only incorrect. Thus, the null hypothesis is put forward that a given scientific manipulation (i.e., drug treatment) will do nothing or have no effect on the receptor system. Then, data is collected to disprove this hypothesis. If the data do not disprove the hypothesis, this does *not* mean that the hypothesis of no difference is correct, because the design of the experiment may simply have been inadequate to show the difference. Therefore, the aim is to design careful experiments to disprove the null hypothesis of no difference and to advance ideas by continually disproving null hypotheses.

Similarly, statistical procedures do not prove anything but merely allow calculation of a probability of acceptance: That is, the analysis may yield a statistic suggesting that there is a 95% certainty that a given hypothesis is unacceptable. However, there is always the 5% chance that the statistic is misleading and, in spite of ones best efforts at experimental design, a hypothesis that should be accepted is wrongly rejected (i.e., the data fall within the 5% chance).

Tables of calculated statistics are available to determine uncertainty; two used in this chapter are the t and the F statistic. From the calculated value of either t or F and comparison to the tables, we can gain a measure of where the dataset lies when it is calculated with different models. In general, a sum of squares (SSq) is calculated that is the sum of the square of the differences of the actual value of each data point (y) and the calculated value of that data point (y_c) according to the following model:

$$SSq = \sum (y - y_c)^2 \qquad [9.1]$$

Models differ in terms of complexity (see Chapter 4). In general, the more fitting constants there are in the equations, the more sensitive they will be to nuances in the data and, therefore, the better will be the fit. However, with each newly added fitting constant, the model becomes less informative; that is, it becomes less clear which parameters are responsible for the changes in the data. In general, less information is gained from more complex models.

Models should be as simple as possible so that differences in datasets can be ascribed to differences in the models. Therefore, if a test for significant difference between a complex and a simple model yields a value for F that is not high enough to support these models' differences, the simpler model should be chosen. The calculation of F from the sum of squares for the simple model [SSq(s)] and the complex model [SSq(c)] is given by:

$$F = \frac{((SSq(c) - SSq(s))(df_s - df_c))}{SSq(c)/df_c} \qquad [9.2]$$

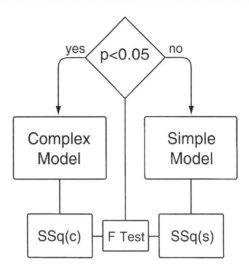

FIGURE 9-2. *Hypothesis testing through the method of increasing sum of squares (SSq). The SSq for the most complex model and the next simplest model are calculated. If the F test shows no significant difference between the two, then the simpler model is preferred. If F is significant at the preselected level (i.e., p = .05), then there is a significant difference between the two models and the more complex model is preferred.*

where *df* refers to the degrees of freedom of the model (determined from various calculations with n, the number of elements in the dataset minus the number of fitting constants). In these circumstances, hypothesis testing becomes a series of comparisons of data to models of increasing simplicity (Fig 9-2). The use of Equation 9.2 will be dealt with specifically in sections on linear and nonlinear fitting of data.

9.4 MEAN AND STANDARD ERROR

The most utilized statistic for central tendency in pharmacology is the mean (or average). Often, datasets comprise two sample means, and the question asked is, "Are they different?" The confidence one has regarding the difference between two means is linked to the magnitude of the variability of the measurement: That is, two means may be numerically very close, but if there is a very low error associated with their measurement, the probability that they will be shown to be different may still be very high. The standard error (SE) of the mean of a sample composed of *x* elements is calculated using the following equation:

$$SE = \left[\frac{n\sum x^2 - (\sum x)^2}{n^2(n-1)} \right]^{1/2}$$

[9.3]

An important statistic, designated t, can be obtained from tables and allows the calculation of confidence when multiplied by the standard error. The value of t varies with the sample size [referred to as the degrees of freedom as calculated by $(n - 1)$]. For example, if the mean of a sample of five estimates of potency for a given agonist (as the pD_2) is 8.5 with a standard error of 0.15, then the following statements about confidence can be made from these values: The value for t with a sample size of 4 [$(5 - 1)$ = 4 degrees of freedom] for a 95% level of confidence ($t_{0.05}$) is 2.76 (obtained from tables). The confidence limit is the value of t multiplied by the standard error, in this case 0.414. What this means is that there is a 95% probability that the true population value for the pK_B from this sample lies between 0.414 less than and greater than the mean or, in this case, there is a 95% probability that the true affinity lies between the values 8.09 and 8.81 (Fig 9-3). Confidence limits are more useful than simple estimates of standard error as they take into account the size of the sample from which the estimate is made.

Confidence limits can be used to assess whether there is a difference between two means. The calculation of the significance statistic t in these circumstances is expressed as follows:

$$t = \frac{x_{m1} - x_{m2}}{sp(1/n_1 + 1/n_2)} \qquad [9.4]$$

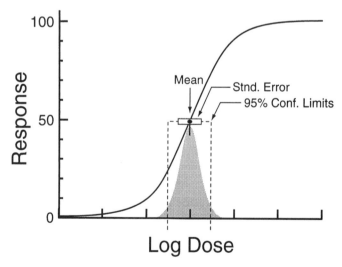

FIGURE 9-3. *Quantification of drug potency (system sensitivity). The mean 50% effective concentration (EC_{50}) is shown, along with the limits of the standard error and the 95% confidence limits. These latter limits set the range between which 95% of all of the estimates of the population should lie.*

where the two means are x_{m1} and x_{m2}, n refers to the number of elements in each sample, and sp is a calculation from the pooled variance given by the following equation:

$$sp^2 = \frac{\sum x_1^2 + \sum x_2^2 - \left(\sum x_1\right)^2/n_1 - \left(\sum x_2\right)^2/n_2}{n_1 + n_2 - 2} \qquad [9.5]$$

Table 9-1 shows six estimates of the potency of two agonists on a receptor system. Equation 9.5 yields an estimate of the pooled variance of 0.051, with a resulting t value for the difference between the two potencies of 2.9. These values of t are compared to values in tables to give the degree of certainty that the difference is real (i.e., the *significance*). The t values for the degrees of freedom (n) for this example are shown at the bottom of Table 9-1. It can be seen that the experimentally derived t is larger than the t value for $p < .025$ but smaller than the t value for $p < .01$. The highest value of t from the tables that is below the experimental t is 2.634 (for $p < 0.025$). What this means is that there is less than a 2.5% chance that the two means are not different. To put this another way, there is a 97.5% chance that the two means are indeed truly different and that the difference did not occur by random chance. The

TABLE 9-1 pD$_2$ (−Log EC$_{50}$) Values for Two Agonists in a Receptor System

Agonist A (x_1)	Agonist B (x_2)	Sums	
8.1	8.1		
8.3	8.1	$\Sigma x_1 = 50.7$	$\Sigma x_2 = 48.3$
8.7	8.4		
8.3	7.9	$\Sigma x_1^2 = 413.6$	$\Sigma x_2^2 = 392.3$
8.1	7.8		
8.3	8.2	$n_1 = n_2 = 6$	
$x_{1m} = 8.30$	$x_{2m} = 8.08$		

Difference between means x and x = 0.22

Standard error of the difference = 0.13

t = 2.9 , p < .025

			t values for 10 degrees of freedom for probability of a larger value					
p < .5	.4	.2	.1	.05	.025	.010	.005	.001
t = 0.7	0.879	1.372	1.812	2.228	2.634	3.169	3.581	4.587

means are different, but there is a 2.5% chance that this is an incorrect conclusion: The investigator must assume the responsibility of judgment and decide whether this degree of uncertainty is acceptable. Note that larger t values are required for a greater degree of certainty to accept that the two means are indeed different. It can be seen from Equation 9.4 that this would result either from a larger difference between the means or from a smaller pooled variance (i.e., more accurate measurement of the two means).

An estimate of the standard error of the difference between the means can be calculated by the following equation:

$$SE_{difference} = [sp^2(1/n_1 + 1/n_2)]^{1/2} \qquad [9.6]$$

For the example shown in Table 9-1, this value is 0.13. Therefore, the difference in potency between the two agonists (in log units) is 0.22 ± 0.13.

9.5 ANALYSIS OF STRAIGHT LINES

Linear representations of data lend themselves to straightforward analysis. The independent variable usually is chosen for the x axis (abscissae) in Cartesian coordinates with the ordinates (y axis) representing the dependent variables. It is assumed that random variability occurs only in values for y. As with nonlinear curve fitting (see Chapter 3), the best-fit straight line is obtained by calculating the square of the distance between the calculated line and the data points (least squares method, Equation 9.1). The sum of these squared deviations (designated SSq) functions as an indicator of the goodness of fit of the data points to the calculated line.

Given a set of y values for designated values of x, the first question to be considered is whether there is a regression of y upon x: That is, does the value of y depend in some way on the value of x? A measure of confidence for this comes from the calculation of the regression coefficient. As an example, Table 9-2 shows the saturation maximal asymptotes for a series of cellular expression systems containing various levels of receptor (x values as counted by an antagonist radioligand in picomoles per milligram of protein). The ordinate y values are the same sites counted with a radioactive agonist (thereby reflecting the number of G-protein bound receptors in the same cells). A number of summations of the x and y values allow the calculation of the regression coefficient m (see Table 9-2). The standard deviation of the regression coefficient is expressed as follows:

$$s_m = \left[\frac{(s_y^2)(s_x^2) - (s_{xy})^2}{(n-2)(s_y^2)^2} \right]^{1/2} \qquad [9.7]$$

TABLE 9-2 Amount of High Affinity of Agonist-Receptor Ternary Complex for Given Expression Levels of Receptors

Antagonist Sites [x (pM/mg)]	Agonist Sites [y (pM/mg)]	$(y - y_p)^2$	Sums	
1.29	0.88	0.018		
1.47	1.31	0.03	$\Sigma x = 52.7$	$\Sigma y = 37.3$
3.41	2.22	0.065	$\Sigma y^2 = 296$	
6.97	5.65	0.51	$\Sigma x^2 = 593$	
11.08	6.55	1.48	$\Sigma (y - yp)^2 = 3.753$	
13.56	10.7	1.49	$\Sigma xy = 416.7$	
14.9	10	0.16	$n = 7$	

$$s_x^2 = \Sigma x^2 - (\Sigma x)^2/n = 196.2 \quad s_y^2 = \Sigma y^2 - (\Sigma y)^2/n = 97.2$$

$$s_{xy} = \Sigma xy - (\Sigma x)(\Sigma y)/n = 135.9$$

$$\text{Regression coefficient} = m = \frac{(\Sigma x)(\Sigma y) - (\Sigma xy)n}{(\Sigma x)^2 - (\Sigma x^2)n}$$

From the regression coefficient and its standard deviation can be calculated a t value to assess the significance of the dependence of y on x:

$$t = m / s_m \ (df = n - 2) \qquad [9.8]$$

For the example shown in Table 9-2, $m = 0.69$ and $s_b = 0.113$. The value of t is 6.1, indicating that there is less than a 0.5% probability that the measured numbers of agonist binding sites occurred by chance and did not depend on the total number of receptors in the preparation. Given this, a straight line can be calculated to represent the dependence, as follows:

$$y = m x + c \qquad [9.9]$$

with m being the slope (calculated in Table 9-2) and c the intercept, given by the following equation:

$$c = \frac{(\Sigma y) - m(\Sigma x)}{n} \qquad [9.10]$$

The data shown in Table 9-2 yield the straight-line fit shown in Figure 9-4A. A measure of how well the data fit the model of a straight line can be gained from calculating the squares of the Ssq (see Equation 9.1).

The error of the various parameters determining straight lines also can be calculated; the equations for these calculations (Equations 9.11–9.15) are given in Table 9-3. The standard error of y is useful for determining the

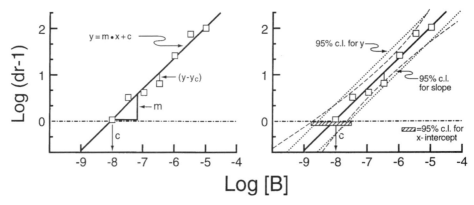

FIGURE 9-4. *Linear regression. A. Data for a Schild analysis (see Chapter 8) plotted as a linear regression. Shown is the best-fit straight line (y = mx + c) and an example of a difference between an actual and calculated data point (y−y$_c$) .The slope is the increase in y for given x (m), and c is the x intercept when y=0. B. Regression shown in A. Curved dotted lines show the 95% confidence limits (c.l.) of the slope; straight dotted lines show the 95% confidence limits for an estimate of y. The hatched horizontal bar shows the 95% confidence limits of a calculated value of x, in this case, the x intercept (pK$_B$).*

TABLE 9-3   Equations for Calculation of Regression Statistics

---

Standard error of the slope

$$SE_m = \left[\frac{n\,SSq}{(n-2)\,[n(\Sigma x^2) - (\Sigma x)^2]} \right]^{1/2} \qquad [9.11]$$

Standard error of the y intercept

$$SE_c = \left[\frac{SSq(\Sigma x^2)}{(n-2)\,[n(\Sigma x^2) - (\Sigma x)^2]} \right]^{1/2} \qquad [9.12]$$

Standard error of y

$$SE_y = \left[\frac{SSq}{(n-2)} \left[\frac{1}{n} + \frac{(x - x_m)^2}{\Sigma x^2} \right] \right]^{1/2} \qquad [9.13]$$

Standard error of predicted y

$$SE_{yc} = \left[\frac{SSq}{(n-2)} \left[1 + \frac{1}{n} + \frac{(x - x_m)^2}{\Sigma x^2} \right] \right]^{1/2} \qquad [9.14]$$

Confidence limits x for calc. x

$$x = \frac{x \pm \dfrac{t}{m} \left[\dfrac{SSq}{(n-2)} \left[\dfrac{n+1}{n} (1 - c)^2 + \dfrac{x_c^2}{\Sigma x^2} \right] \right]^{1/2}}{1 - c^2} \qquad [9.15]$$

where $c = \dfrac{t^2\,SSq\Sigma x^2}{(n-2)(\Sigma xy)^2}$

confidence limits of the calculated line (c.f. $= \pm t \times SE_y$; see Fig 9-4B). Similarly, the confidence limits for any calculated value of y for a given value of x can be obtained with the SE_{yc} (Equation 9.14; see Fig 9-4B). For the process of linear calibration, the regression line may be used to interpolate or extrapolate a value of x (see Fig 9-4B). The 95% confidence limits of the x value from this process are given by Equation 9.15.

Straight lines can differ from one another by slope or location along the x axis. There are numerous instances when a difference in slope of lines is an important factor in the choice of drug-receptor models. The datasets may simply represent two lines (individually having slopes m_1 and m_2) with the same slope but different locations (i.e., a parallel shift in the line). In these circumstances, the common slope (m_c) can be calculated:

$$m_c = \frac{W_1 m_1 + W_2 m_2}{W_1 + W_2}$$ [9.16]

where W_1 and W_2 are weighting factors, the magnitudes of which are inversely proportional to the standard errors of the individual slopes:

$$W = (1/SE_m)^2$$ [9.17]

The best-fit straight line of the data points with a common slope then is given by:

$$y = y_m + m_c(x - x_m)$$ [9.18]

where y_m and x_m refer to the mean of y and x respectively.

An example of how these equations can be used is provided in the models that follow. Figure 9-5 shows two datasets comprising the number of expressed receptors in a collection of stable cell lines and their corresponding number of high-affinity binding sites for agonist, referring to the number of receptor-G-protein couples that can be formed with a high-efficacy agonist radioligand. The two datasets represent the wild-type receptor and a site-directed mutant of the same receptor. Differences between the relationship of receptor number and high-affinity complex number can be interpreted as differences in the behavior of the mutant toward the G-protein. The question asked is: "Did site-directed mutagenesis alter the behavior of the receptor toward the G-protein?" This question can be approached by the principle of extra sum of squares. The data are subjected to fitting to three models of differing complexity. The first and most complex (and therefore, most easily fit) is the model of two lines of differing slope and intercept (model 1):

$$\text{Model 1}$$
$$y_1 = m_1 x + c_1$$
$$y_2 = m_2 x + c_2$$ [9.19]

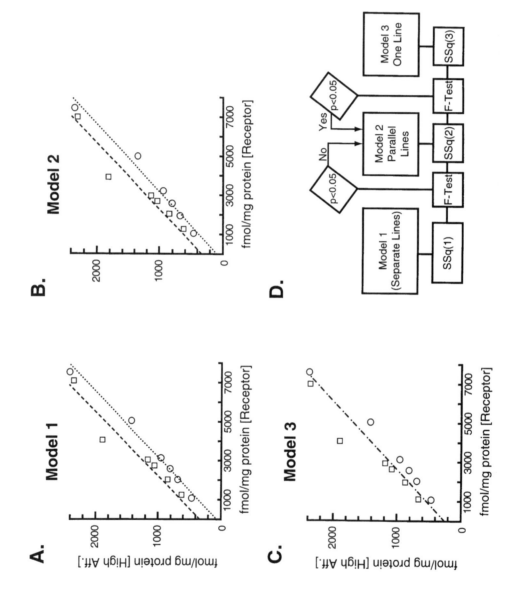

The second, and simpler, model is one of differing location parameters (intercepts) but common slope (model 2; see Fig 9-5B):

Model 2

$$y_1 = mx + c_1$$
$$y_2 = mx + c_2 \qquad\qquad [9.20]$$

The common slope is calculated using Equation 9.17 and the line using Equation 9.10. Now the statistic F for preference of one model over the other can be calculated according to Equation 9.2. Model 1 is the most complex; thus the SSq for this will be termed SSq(c). Model 2 (common slope) is simpler [SSq(s)]. The degrees of freedom equal the sum of the number of elements in each dataset ($n_1 + n_2$) minus the number of constant parameters. Model 1 has four fitting constants (m_1, m_2, c_1, c_2); therefore, the $df_1 = 8$. Model 2 has three fitting constants (m, c_1, c_2) therefore, the $df = 9$. The resulting values for the sum of squares from the example shown in Figure 9-5 are shown in Table 9-4. The value of F ($F = 0.107$) indicates that the change from model 1 to model 2 is not statistically significant; therefore, the simpler model (2) is preferred. The next step is to compare the data to an even simpler model, in which both datasets fit to a single straight line (Fig 9-5C):

Model 3

$$y = mx + c \qquad\qquad [9.21]$$

The degrees of freedom for this model is derived thus: $n_1 + n_2 - 2$. The calculation (shown in Table 9-4) indicates that the value of F ($F = 5.48$) is significant at the 95% level (i.e., there is a less than 5% probability that the difference between models 2 and 3 could have occurred by chance). Therefore, model 2 is preferred over model 3. The analysis indicates that the dataset is best fit by two parallel straight lines (i.e., that the point mutation caused a difference in the behavior of the receptor toward G-proteins). The complete sequence of hypothesis testing for these sets of data is shown schematically in Figure 9-5D.

FIGURE 9-5. *Comparison of two regression lines. Data showing the amount of high-affinity binding complex for an agonist radioligand as a function of the expressed receptor number for a wild-type receptor (circles) and a site-directed mutant receptor (squares). A. Model 1 fits the data points to two separate lines with separate slopes and intercepts. B. Model 2 fits the data to two separate but parallel straight lines. C. Model 3 fits the two datasets to a single straight line. D. These various models were subjected to the F test. The sequence shows that the F test did not exhibit significant difference between model 1 and model 2; therefore, model 2 (the simpler of the two) was chosen and tested against model 3. The F test for this comparison showed significant difference, therefore, model 2 was chosen overall.*

TABLE 9-4 Extra Sum of Squares for Regression Lines (data from Fig 9-5)

Model 1

(two lines with different slopes and intercepts)

Wild-type receptor	$y = 0.299x + 62.18$
Site-directed mutant	$y = 0.314x + 280.7$

SSq = 1,072,020; df = 8

Model 2

(two lines of common slope but different intercepts)

Wild-type receptor	$y = 0.3x + 61$
Site-directed mutant	$y = 0.3x + 329.2$

SSq = 1,057,659; df = 9

Model 3

(data fit to single line)

Both receptors	$y = 0.3x + 186$

SSq = 413,035; df = 10

9.6 POPULATION ANALYSIS

If a sample dataset is homogenous then the frequency of values will form a normal bell-shaped curve along the axis of standard error (Fig 9-6A). The area under the curve represents the amount of the dataset being considered. Therefore, if a dataset were large enough, it could be divided into bins representing frequency, and these frequencies would form a histogram that resembled a normal curve (Fig 9-6B). Practically speaking, datasets usually are not large enough to gain a measure of their normality (symmetry along the axis of the mean), and the number of populations seldom is clear from histograms (compare Fig 9-6B and Fig 9-6C).

If these areas were to be plotted as a function of logarithms of the data points, then a sigmoidal curve would result. For example, Figure 9-7A shows straight vertical lines cutting the area under the bell-shaped curve at 10%, 20%, 30%, 40%, 50%, and 80%. Figure 9-7B shows the sigmoidal curve resulting from plotting the cumulative area for given values of the dataset. Such sigmoidal curves can be useful for analyzing single or multiple populations. Very often the question is asked: "Does a particular drug treatment alter the responsiveness of a biologic preparation?" If the answer is yes, then two samples of data

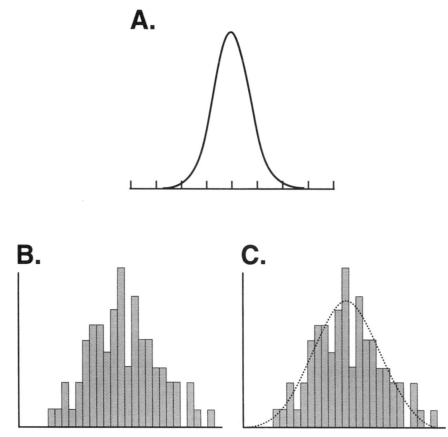

FIGURE 9-6. *Distributions as histograms. A. A theoretical single population distribution of estimates. B. An experimental sample of estimates grouped and plotted as a frequency distribution histogram. C. Comparison of a single-population theoretical distribution on the experimental distribution. It is not clear from the histogram whether one or two populations of samples are present in the dataset.*

composed of drug-treated and untreated biologic responses should arise from different populations and therefore be discernible with population analysis. As seen in Figure 9-7B, a single population results in a simple single-phase sigmoidal curve. As two populations differ with respect to their mean or size, the resulting cumulative frequency curve takes on a biphasic shape (Fig 9-8A to D). These multiphases can be modeled mathematically with equations and the fit of the data points tested with nonlinear curve-fitting techniques. Thus, a cumulative frequency curve can be fit by models depicting single and multiple populations, and a statistical test of significance can be conducted to determine the probability of single or multiple populations. As for linear regression analysis, the principle of extra sum of squares can be used. The cumulative frequency curve for the dataset shown in Figure 9-6 is shown in Figure 9-9. In Figure 9-9A, the best-fit single-population cumulative frequency curve is shown; the data do

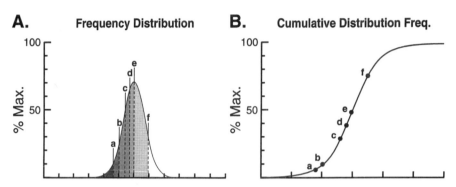

FIGURE 9-7. *Conversion of a distribution to a cumulative frequency curve. A. A distribution for a dataset; the area under the curve represents various proportions of the population. Points a to f show sections of area under the curve increasing from left to right (cutoff a represents the area from the left end of the curve to the line denoted by a, cutoff f represents the area from the left end of the curve to the line denoted by f, etc.). B. The cumulative areas as ordinate values on a curve plotted against the values present in the population. The areas from left to right across the distribution, when added together, form a sigmoidal curve, which then can be analyzed for heterogeneity in a manner similar to that used for the detection of heterogeneous receptor populations.*

not fit the model. In contrast, a two-population cumulative frequency model provides an adequate fit of the dataset (Fig 9-9B).

9.7 NONLINEAR REGRESSION (SINGLE-PHASE OR MULTIPHASE CURVES)

In general, it is better to use nontransformed data for analysis (without a mathematic process to convert the data from a curved line to a straight line) if possible. With the advent of computer fitting of data to complex models, this can easily be done. It is useful to fit the dataset to the minimal model (least number of parameters). One of the most frequently asked questions in pharmacology relates to the homogeneity of a population of receptors. As discussed in Chapter 3, the Langmuir adsorption isotherm is a useful model for the binding of drugs to a homogeneous single population of receptor sites. The result is a monophasic sigmoidal binding curve representing a normal population of binding sites. Deviation from this model may represent a mixture of binding sites (receptors) which, in turn, may be a useful and therapeutically advantageous situation. As binding occurs to mixed populations, deviations from a monophasic sigmoidal curve are observed. These deviations vary with the relative size and separation of the populations with respect to sensitivity to the drug (i.e., see curves in Fig 9-8). The principle of increased sum of squares can be used to test datasets for single or multiple phases. For example, Figure 9-10A shows a saturation binding curve of a

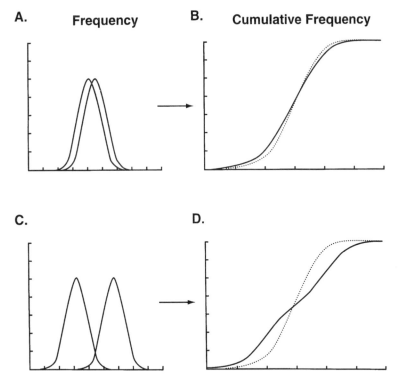

FIGURE 9-8. *Dual populations represented by cumulative frequency curves. A. Two closely related populations. B. The cumulative curve for the two populations together. The dotted line represents the cumulative frequency curve for a single population. The deviation between the two curves indicates the presence of two populations. C. Two more widely diverging populations. D. The cumulative frequency curve for the populations shown in C. It can be seen that the cumulative frequency curve for the data clearly diverges from a single-population curve (dotted line).*

radioligand to a receptor system. The data can be fit to a three-receptor-site model, the equation for which is:

$$y = \frac{37[A]}{[A] + 0.0137} + \frac{39.3[A]}{[A] + 0.67} + \frac{26[A]}{[A] + 0.72} \qquad [9.22]$$

This can be considered a model of high complexity (six fitting constants). The SSq for these data is 737.838 with 38 degrees of freedom ($n - 6$). The same dataset then can be fit to a model of two populations of binding sites and a value of F calculated (Equation 9.2) to determine statistical significance. Thus, the same dataset can be fit to the following equation:

$$y = \frac{37[A]}{[A] + 0.013} + \frac{63[A]}{[A] + 0.69} \qquad [9.23]$$

The SSq for this model is 737.78 ($df = n-4= 40$). The calculated F for the difference between these models is 0.004, which is not significant.

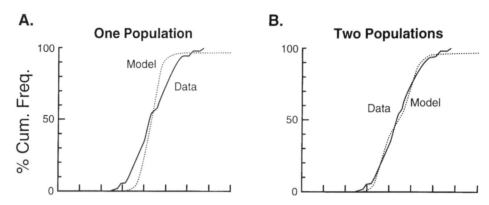

FIGURE 9-9. *Cumulative frequency curve for histogram data shown in Figure 9-6B. A. The data clearly differ from a single-population model (dotted line). B. The data can be fit to a model made up of two populations. These data suggest that the histogram is a sampling from a two-population dataset.*

Therefore, this test indicates that there is no difference between the complex three-population model and the simpler two-population model. In these circumstances, the simplest model is preferred. The process then can be repeated for a single population model. The best-fit single-population model is given by the following equation:

$$y = \frac{98.4\,[A]}{[A] + 0.16} \qquad [9.24]$$

As can be seen from Figure 9-10B, the data fit poorly to this model, and an *F* test shows a high degree of statistical significance between the two-population and the single-population model. Therefore, the dataset is best fit by a model depicting two populations of binding sites.

These data also illustrate a fallacy of curve fitting as apparent proof of hypothesis. The same data points can be fit to models of numerous populations of binding sites. Figure 9-10C shows the calculated line for a three-population model (according to Equation 9.22) and for a two-population model (according to Equation 9.23). It can be seen that these are nearly identical. Moreover, a model of four or more populations would indicate a similar curve. This shows that the shape of a dose-response curve cannot be used as proof of a molecular mechanism. However, the converse—namely, that a predicted shape of a curve from a model must mimic the data—is a prerequisite for acceptance of a model.

9.8 EXPERIMENTAL DESIGN

Many factors control the power of the testing, and only a few are under the experimenter's control. These are the significance level chosen to base differ-

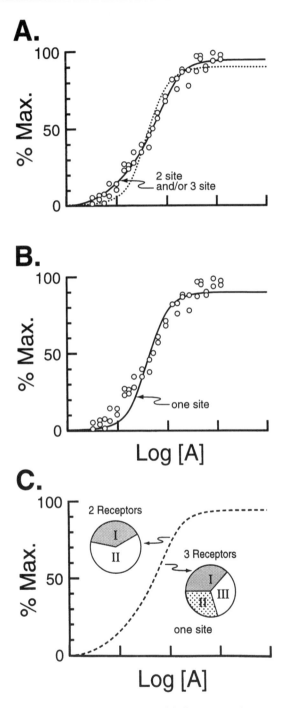

FIGURE 9-10. *Receptor binding data. A. Data can be fit to models for two- or three-receptor populations according to Equations 9.23 and 9.22, respectively. B. The data points diverge significantly from a single-receptor population model. C. Note how the complex curve fitting the data is nearly identical for the two- and the three-receptor model, illustrating the fallacy of using the shape of the binding curve to infer the exact number of populations.*

ence, the sample size (n) and, sometimes, the range of elements chosen for the sample. This latter factor can be important in linear regression, in which the slope of the line is an important determinant of the acceptance of the estimate (i.e., slopes for Schild regressions different from unity do not furnish molecular estimates of antagonist potency) and also, in which parameters are extrapolated from calculated lines. Figure 9-11 shows two Schild regressions for an antagonist, one calculated from a wide range of dose ratios and another from a narrow range of dose ratios. As can be seen from the 95% confidence limits of the slope, the narrow range is much more variable, leading to a less useful estimate of the pK_B. Clearly, for Schild regression, the larger the range of dose ratios, the better the estimate of the slope and the pK_B.

Another instance in which this arises is in the detection of responses or receptor signals in expression cloning studies. The genetic expression of re-

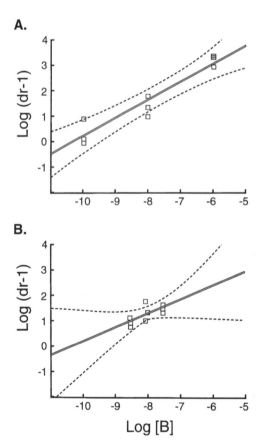

FIGURE 9-11. *The effect of the range of data on the resulting estimation of parameters. A. A Schild regression obtained from a wide range of dose ratios (dr). The dotted lines represent the 95% confidence limits on the slope of the regression. B. A Schild regression from a small range of dose ratios. The variance of the slope (rotation about the mean x and y) is very high because there are no data points to limit the variance on the ends of the regression.*

ceptors and other biologic materials in cells is quickly becoming one of the most important types of stop-time experiments in pharmacology. This work represents the proverbial search for a "needle in a haystack," in that only a small fraction of the transiently expressed cells contain expressed receptors. Much of this is a random process in that a large collection of cDNA fragments is introduced into a milieu of cells. Only one of those cells may take in the correct cDNA and express the complete and operable population of receptors, and this cell must be detected in the population of cells that have no operable receptor. The process of screening for the cell or cells that have the correctly assembled and expressed receptor uses a label for that receptor. The dependent variable readout may be a response (as in oocyte electrophysiologic response) or radiolabel binding.

This process becomes another sampling problem in that only a few cells in the colony must be detected, and so there are no replicate samples, and no concentration range of detecting drug can be used. There are theoretic and practical reasons for choosing a concentration of detecting drug that should produce the maximal signal. Figure 9-12A shows a hypothetical dataset of the dose-response curve for expressed receptors in a foci of 20 cells. The data have been constructed such that the maximal asymptote (i.e., receptor expression level) and the location of the dose-response curve (i.e., sensitivity of the cell to labeling drug) have been subjected to random error by computer. Figure 9-12B shows the mean with standard errors of the mean of the 20 curves. It also shows the standard error of the measurement at each level of signal, expressed as a percentage of the signal. In general, this simulation shows that a maximal dose of detecting ligand should be used (balanced against the possible nonspecific effects of such a high dose).

Another possible control in experimentation is the sample size. Because statistical significance depends on n, calculations can be made to yield the n for a required degree of certainty and accuracy. Under these circumstances, n is expressed thus:

$$n = \left[\frac{t\sigma}{E} \right]^2 \qquad [9.25]$$

where E is the maximal error that will be tolerable, t the value for significance, and σ the standard error of the population. For instance, suppose that the potency of a given antagonist will be used to determine the nature of a receptor and that a 95% confidence limit will be used to determine significance ($t = 1.96$). Normal estimates of pK_B vary approximately threefold (on a log scale, this sets σ at 0.47). To allow a maximal error of twofold difference in the estimated potency to make this assessment, a sample value of $[(1.96)(0.47)/(0.3)^2] = 9$ will be required. These types of calculations are useful in experimental design.

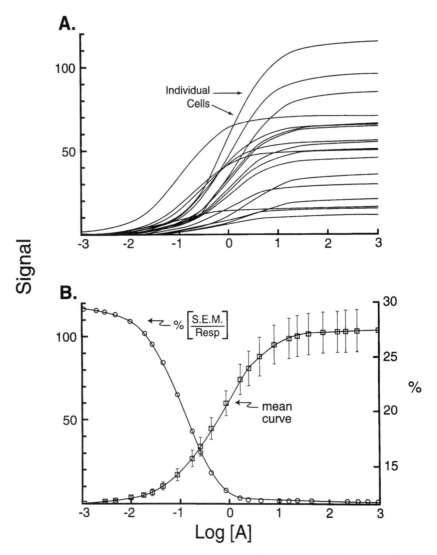

FIGURE 9-12. *Expression cloning data for 40 transiently expressed cells in a population. A. The dose-response curves to an agonist in 40 cells is shown with random variation on receptor expression level and sensitivity to the radioligand. B. The mean of the curves is shown with standard errors of the means (SEM). The standard error, as a function of the signal strength, is illustrated as well. With the higher doses of the radioligand, the signal-to-noise ratio is minimal (i.e., a high dose of radioligand is best to detect the signal).*

There are numerous sources of error in measurement, and the overall significance of a finding often is simply a question of "signal-to-noise" ratio. As discussed in other parts of this book, there are statistical and methodologic ways to deal with this problem and it should be possible to make valid scientific observations that spawn illumination and insight. However, in addition to this, the introduction of "*fuzzy logic*" enters in many biologic questions and theoretically can influence the path of research. This specialized term refers to the handling of datasets that defy definitive classification. As the complexity of a system, such as a cell, increases, the ability to make precise statements about this system decreases until a situation emerges in which relevance and precision become mutually exclusive characteristics. Three sources of uncertainty in science are *errors in measurement* (i.e., incomplete resolution), *random errors,* and a type of error that involves fuzzy logic datasets—namely, *linguistic imprecision.* This latter source of error enters into all realms of biologic classification, especially in the subclassification of receptors. In general, a receptor subtype invites vague concepts, inferences, and rules.

A major consideration in receptor biology is the making of a physiologic conclusion from numeric data. This is done by accumulating enough data to show a clear statistical difference. Figure 9-13 shows pK_i values for six antagonists on four receptors obtained in surrogate cell lines by expression cloning. It is not known whether the receptors are identical or are, in fact, splice variants of the same receptor gene. Therefore, it is relevant to correlate pharmacologic profiles of antagonists to determine similar behaviors. If all possible correlations of these datasets are made, it is apparent that there are no data to classify receptors I, III, and VI as being different from one another (i.e., the existing data show no divergence in potencies). As discussed in Chapter 1, this still does not constitute adequate data to classify the receptors as being the same, as the antagonists that show a difference may not have been tested. However, the dataset clearly furnishes data to support the conclusion that receptors II, IV, and V differ.

Another potential problem comes in partially correlating datasets. For example, if one considers the universe of red apples and not-red apples, where does one classify a half-red and half-green apple? In receptor biology, this has the usual outcome of considering a receptor as "subtype X-like." The pK_i profiles for two receptors with eight antagonists is shown in Table 9-5. Though seven of the estimates correlate very well, one (*E* in the table) shows a clear difference. Such datasets have been used to classify receptors as "Receptor X-like," but there are hazards in such classifications. With such a linguistic classification, the expectation is that further testing of drugs selective for receptor X will also be active on the new X-like receptor, an expectation for which there is no support. The data showing a difference in potency disproves the null hypothesis of no difference between the two receptors, and so they must be considered different biologic entities. However, this would not preclude medicinal chemists from using receptor X templates to make drugs for the X-like receptor. Another question raised by such data is the choice of reclassifying the system (receptor) or the drug. The fact that one drug stands out from the seven others may mean either that it is the one that

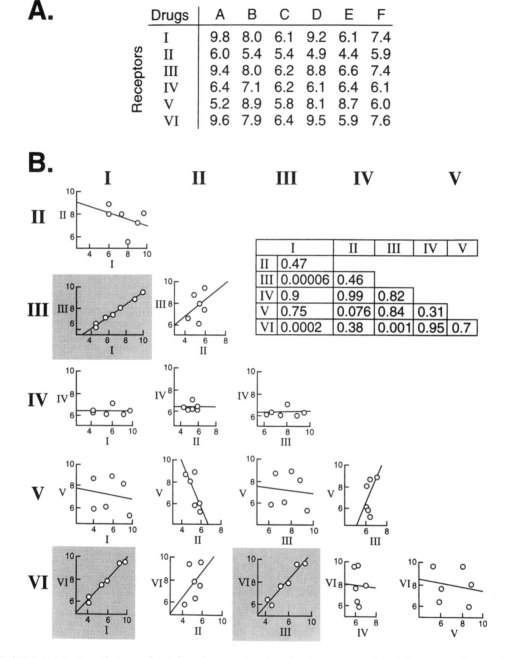

A.

Receptors \ Drugs	A	B	C	D	E	F
I	9.8	8.0	6.1	9.2	6.1	7.4
II	6.0	5.4	5.4	4.9	4.4	5.9
III	9.4	8.0	6.2	8.8	6.6	7.4
IV	6.4	7.1	6.2	6.1	6.4	6.1
V	5.2	8.9	5.8	8.1	8.7	6.0
VI	9.6	7.9	6.4	9.5	5.9	7.6

B.

	I	II	III	IV	V
II	0.47				
III	0.00006	0.46			
IV	0.9	0.99	0.82		
V	0.75	0.076	0.84	0.31	
VI	0.0002	0.38	0.001	0.95	0.7

FIGURE 9-13. *Correlations of pK$_i$ data for receptor classification. A. The pK$_i$ of six antagonists on six receptors is shown. Identical receptors should show identical pK$_i$ profiles. B. Correlations of each of the receptors in terms of the pK$_i$ profiles. Most correlations are poor but it can be seen that correlations of I to III, I to VI, and III to VI are reasonable. The inset table shows the significance levels for the correlations shown. The fact that the corresponding significance levels for these correlations are 0.00006, 0.0002, and 0.001, respectively (this quantifies the percentage of probability that the correlations arose by chance and are not real), indicates that receptors I, III, and VI form a related set (i.e., they could be the same receptor type).*

TABLE 9-5 Correlations of Pk$_i$ Values on Two Receptor Systems with Eight Drugs

Drug (pK$_i$)	Receptor I	Receptor II
A	9.7	9.5
B	7.1	6.9
C	8.9	8.7
D	9.2	9.15
E	**6.5**	**7.6**
F	10.1	10.3
G	8.2	8.2
H	7.4	7.2

distinguishes between the two receptors, or that it has another obfuscating property that expresses itself in one system but not the other.

An illustration of further potential problems with classification involves Zeno's Paradox which, simply stated, is: "When is a heap of sand not a heap of sand?" If one has a heap of sand and defines it as such, then does the removal of one grain take it out of this classification or is it still a heap of sand? This continues: Does the removal of two grains of sand, three grains, or more void this classification? At what point are enough grains removed that another classification becomes acceptable (i.e., it is no longer a heap of sand; see Fig 9-14)? The problem lies in the subjectivity of these classifications; one observer may consider that the sand is no longer a heap before another concludes this because each has different classification standards. Thus, a fuzzy dataset exists.

The fuzziness of the data may depend on the vantage point from which it is viewed. For example, the pK_i profiles shown in Figure 9-12 may suggest that receptors I, III, and VI are not different, but they may assume that an amino acid sequence analysis indicates that the amino acid sequences of receptors I and II are identical and that some amino acids in receptor III are different. This closer look would constitute evidence to show that receptor III was indeed different from receptors I and II. However, the constellation of amino acid protein conformations cannot be accounted for and, however unlikely it may seem, it still may be that the cellular host of receptor I induces a different tertiary conformation than that for receptor II in its host, thereby precluding identity in their respective hosts. Thus, as the magnifying glass of inspection gains power, the vantage point for Zeno's paradox changes and so too does the conclusion of difference.

Zeno's Paradox

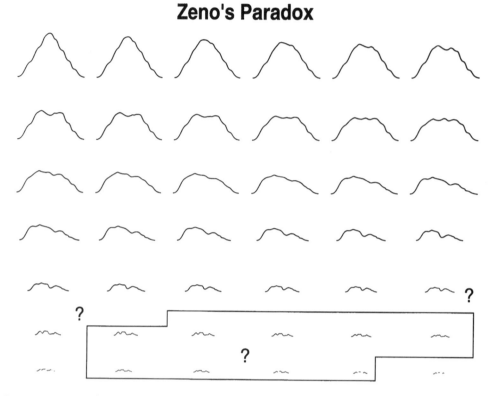

FIGURE 9-14. *Zeno's paradox: "When is a heap of sand not a heap of sand?" As consecutive single grains of sand are removed from the pile, soon there is a gray area (shown by the area within the boxed outline) where some dubiety exists: Are these different from the preceding piles or smaller versions of the same? Similar questions are raised in the classification of receptors when profiles resemble each other but do not exactly match.*

9.9 SYNOPSIS

The following ideas were presented in this chapter:

- Statistics is the study of dispersion and central tendency in data in samples. From these samples, inferences can be made about the populations from which the data originated. Statistics can aid in the definition of signal-to-noise ratio and thus can differentiate real effects from random events.

- Sampling should be as random as possible to represent the population best.

- Models are chosen on the basis of the magnitude of the sum of squares of the deviations between the calculated and experimental values. If the F statistic shows no significant difference between two models, the simplest model is preferred.

- Differences between two sample means can be assessed by calculating a standard error and appropriate confidence limit for difference. The confidence limit is preferred as it incorporates the size of the sample.

- Data that can be assessed in straight-line regressions can be fit to a variety of models from single straight lines to single parallel straight lines to one straight line. Differences in biologic behavior can be inferred from the choice of model found statistically.

- Multiple populations can be assessed by curve fitting to cumulative frequency curves, much like analysis of multiple binding sites. Data can be fit to a number of models, which indicates that a fit to a model does not necessarily imply that the model is an accurate molecular representation of the system.

- Some factors under an experimenter's control are the sample size, the level of significance for acceptance of difference, and the range of independent variables used to collect data. Control of some of these factors can aid in experimental design.

- Linguistic imprecision plays a role in the classification of drugs and receptors, in that sometimes the quality of the data is insufficient to classify receptors and drugs into clear categories.

FURTHER READING

Armitage P. Statistical methods in medical research, 5th ed. Oxford: Blackwell Scientific, 1980.

Box GEP, Hunter WG, Hunter JS. Statistics for experimenters. New York: Wiley, 1978.

Colquhoun D. Lectures in biostatistics. Oxford: Clarendon, 1971.

Cox DR. Planning of experiments. New York: Wiley, 1992.

Finney DJ. Experimental design and its statistical basis. Chicago: University of Chicago Press, 1955.

Snedecor GW, Cochran WG. Statistical methods. Ames, IA: Iowa State University Press, 1979.

INDEX